A CROWN OF THORNS

Surgeons Ishrat Syed and Kalpana Swaminathan write together as Kalpish Ratna. Their book *The Secret Life of Zika Virus* (2017) examined the emergence of Congenital Zika Syndrome. Their newest book is *Synapse* (2019).

KALPISH RATNA

A CROWN OF THORNS

THE CORONAVIRUS AND US

context

cntxt

First published by Context, an imprint of Westland Publications Private Limited, in 2020

1st Floor, A Block, East Wing, Plot No. 40, SP Infocity, Dr MGR Salai, Perungudi, Kandanchavadi, Chennai 600096

Westland, the Westland logo, Context and the Context logo are trademarks of Westland Publications Private Limited, or its affiliates.

ISBN: 9789389648423

10 9 8 7 6 5 4 3 2 1

Typeset by SÜRYA, New Delhi

Printed at Manipal Technologies Limited, Manipal

'What is your substance, whereof are you made,
That millions of strange shadows on you tend?'

– William Shakespeare, *Sonnet 53*,
The Quarto of 1609

'hic incipit pestis'

– John Bretchgirdle, vicar of the Holy Trinity Church, Stratford-upon-Avon, recorded the death of a weaver, Oliver Gunn, on 11 July 1564 in his parish register. 'Here begins the plague' is scribbled in Latin next to the burial entry. This parish register also records the baptism of '*Gulielmus filius Johannes Shakspere*' on 26 April 1564

Contents

1
Why?

All I have is a voice
To undo the folded lie ...
– W.H. Auden, 'September 1, 1939',
from *Another Time*, 1940

Why this book? In the deluge of information about COVID-19 swamping the planet, why would anyone want more?

This plethora is the very reason.

Standing apart from that stampede, this pandemic looks different—and I'd like to share my view. I've been staring at it for a while now. For twenty years, give or take a few, I've looked at epidemics across time.

It began quite by accident.

A doctor's life follows a familiar trajectory. The first five years go in consolidating what you've learnt into what you do. The next ten, over in a blink, are spent in enjoying what you do. That ends in either smugness or resentment. I chose the second. Doing the same things over and over again was irritating, and I had begun to question the tenets of my craft.

By the beginning of this new millennium, the antibiotic era was long over. Puzzled by any number of new diseases, and familiar diseases turned unfamiliar, we plodded well-trodden paths that led, however tortuously, to the blank wall. And there we stopped, banging our heads against it.

This realisation quarrelled with my other life.

A writer's life is sustained by surprise. One never knows what awaits, verso. One is constantly seeking a different point of view.

So, I refused the blank wall.

I looked at the vista of disease in my own city. I examined a brief but tumultuous time in Bombay: the 400 years after European contact, from 1500 to 1900. Through the horrific Victorian years, when epidemics alternated with famines, there emerged a pattern I could not ignore: every epidemic emerged after a drastic change in the environment. *Assault* may be a better word than *change*.

Some epidemics, like cholera, showed a clear timeline of emergence.

But that clarity confused prevalent notions. Notions prevalent when cholera emerged in the Bay of Bengal in 1816 were still prevalent when it emerged in Haiti in 2010. Since the 1990s, we have known that the cholera germ exists in zooplankton in all natural water bodies, especially estuaries. Yet the 2010 Haiti emergence was blamed on contagion from Nepali health workers. Cholera will remain, once and forever, the 'Asiatic' cholera.

Prejudice hampers science. In the midst of a pandemic, science must constantly introspect to clear the slate of presumption and prejudice.

The past is over, I thought, and turned my attention to the now. I looked at how the island on which I live had changed shape in the last fifty years. Once full of hills, it is now flat land. Once full of rivers, it now has just one, a smear of filth entrapped in concrete. Once renowned for its forests and gardens, it is now bereft of trees. In the heart of the metropolis, we have a patch of wilderness that is constricted every day by human habitation. Leopards stroll out occasionally.

The present pandemic reminds me of an incident one hot afternoon about twenty years ago. I was walking home when I grew aware of a rustling that seemed to keep pace with me. I slowed down, and so did it. I hurried, and it stepped up its pace. It seemed to come from the ditch alongside the road. I think we decided on confrontation at the same moment, because there was a kind of breathless hush when we both stopped. We stared at each other, passing swiftly from shock to curiosity, in mutual survey. Just as swiftly, the moment passed, and the pangolin burrowed deeper into the ditch and went its way. It was my first pangolin, and I was probably its first human.

The wild is never far away; we just don't see it. We push into it, grabbing land and water and air. We have moved in on the wild, and for a while now, the wild has moved in on us. Just how much more will it take for us to notice?

The standard narrative of COVID-19 is biased—the virus gets all the attention. But COVID-19 isn't about the virus. *It is about us.*

We are a species in an evolutionary cul-de-sac. The virus is much older at this game of survival. Still, we've survived viruses ever since we emerged, haven't we?

Why then are we on the edge of being the most threatened species on the planet as viruses menace us with strange illnesses every year?

What makes us a doomed population?

History is the narrative of conquest. Disease is the narrative of defeat. Poised between these two, in the midst of a pandemic we seem to be clueless about, I pitch this book as a narrative of hope.

I invite you to take a second look at COVID-19. This time, from a different point of view.

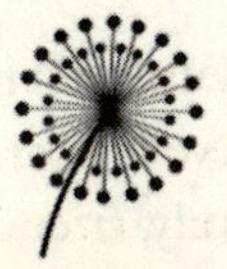

2
The Wuhan Index

... any man's death diminishes me,
because I am involved in mankind.
And therefore never send to know for whom
the bell tolls; it tolls for thee.

– John Donne, 'Meditation XVII',
from *Devotions upon Emergent Occasions*, 1624

Three people in Wuhan, whose names we don't know, are now memorialised in clinical records.

It is from their experience of illness that the world has learnt of COVID-19. A new virus, SARS-CoV-2, isolated from their bodies, inaugurated this pandemic.

Little is known about them. The two who survived must, by now, have told their stories a million times.

In any new disease, the core of understanding is built on the first encounter.

That day must have seemed like any other in the busy outpatients' department of the hospital, its corridors an open textbook of common ailments.

In the months that followed, anybody who was there that day would have returned restlessly to that memory, sifted it for some telltale incident, some detail squirrelled away, something unusual, now bookmarked as prescience or augury. *I was there the very day it all began ...*

December 27, 2019

It was a busy time in Wuhan. There was a frisson in the air; Chūn Jié, the Lunar New Year, was a week ahead. They would be here soon—family, friends, faces missed all year—

was there time enough to prepare comforts, delicacies, treats? People hurried about in anxiety. Shoppers squinted critically at stuff they would have bought without a thought yesterday. Nothing but the best would do today, and the price really wasn't a concern. Not now, not at New Year.

The three people who concern us weren't thinking of the New Year. They worked in the same market, but that was something they would learn afterwards.

In the Wuhan Jinyintan Hospital corridor, in the null hour of waiting, they were strangers.

Patient 1 was a forty-nine-year-old woman. I will name her Guan-Yin, for the Goddess of Mercy.

Guan-Yin peered about nervously and huddled deeper into her jacket. It wasn't as cold as it had been the past few days, but she shivered, nonetheless. At the movement, her daughter placed a light hand against her cheek, and withdrew it, reassured. Guan-Yin nodded. Her fever had let up, but she felt worse, somehow. There was a faint sheen of sweat on her brow, the clammy chill of exhaustion.

'All you need is a good night's rest,' her daughter murmured.

Guan-Yin didn't reply. It made her furious, this reassurance. She didn't want to be told she was fine. She was ill, and she demanded notice.

'It's just the cough keeping you up all night,' the girl continued, her eyes wide with fear.

It tired her to speak, so Guan-Yin merely nodded. How close it was in here, how stale this air! She wanted to break free of her clothes and run out into the sharp cold, to dare its slap on her skin. It would make her gasp and fill her chest with a great big gulp of air. Now, she had to be content with sips. Like a butterfly, she thought, a small, silky-blue butterfly …

Patient 2, a sixty-one-year-old man, stared with sullen curiosity at Guan-Yin because he had to stare at something to stifle his terror. I shall call him Jiān, the sound of flowing water.

Sunk in his coat, Jiān's chest felt as though it would burst any minute. If he concentrated on something—anything—perhaps it would behave till his turn came.

There were three people ahead of him in the queue. What if he couldn't wait? What if he were to fold up right here, slump in this chair, drool, slide to the floor? He scowled angrily.

Guan-Yin, catching his eye, looked hastily away. Her movement made Jiān conscious of his gaffe. He lowered his eyes, embarrassed. When he looked up again, he felt the woman's eyes on his face. She had intelligent eyes. They looked past the opacity of her own suffering, into his. In that instant, they were strangers no more.

Jiān became aware of the young man at his elbow. The daze that gripped him made it difficult to grasp what the fellow was saying. He had noticed the boy earlier, a restless slapdash character. Jobless, probably. And now he had the temerity to demand something. What was he saying? Really, he was most insistent—

The voice formed words at last.

'Can you walk? Let's go in; you can't sit here any longer.'

What a rough voice for such kind words—Jiān shook his head.

This young man, **Patient 3**—I'll call him Bohai, an inlet from the sea—realised the older man felt too weak to walk, and took his hand. Jiān flinched. The young man's hand was red hot.

'You're sicker than me,' Jiān mumbled. 'Get ahead of me in the queue.'

Bohai, thirty-two, stood up with an impatient grumble. He pushed open the clinic door and returned a moment later with an attendant. Jiān found himself being helped into a wheelchair. It was all beyond him now. He glanced again towards the woman with intelligent eyes. She did not disappoint. It was the last thing Jiān noticed before he blacked out—that calm encouragement in her eyes.

Bohai was tired. He leant against the wall, too restless to go back to his seat. This was his third day away from work—wait, hadn't he seen that lady at the market too?

Guan-Yin, too, recognised the young man that very instant. He worked at the Huanan Seafood Market too. And ill, by his flushed look. As if in greeting, both of them coughed.

Neither of them knew, then, that they had something more in common.

We know that all three were hospitalised. We have clinical details that they do not know.

Guan-Yin's chest X-ray has shadows suggestive of a developing pneumonia. Her cough worsens. She breathes oxygen in greedily. Her blood shows a likely viral infection. Her throat is swabbed for testing. Her sputum is spirited away preciously in capped vials.

Jiān cannot breathe. His chest barely moves. He is rapidly losing effort. Things happen very quickly—a tube is passed into his trachea and he's on a ventilator now. The cramped lines on his face have eased. He looks peaceful. Too peaceful.

His lung scan is total chaos. The lungs are webbed, almost solid.

The diagnosis on his case sheet reads: ARDS.

Just a string of letters, an acronym for—what? Another Severe Acute Respiratory Syndrome (SARS)?

Jiān no longer struggles. The machine no longer oxygenates his brain. His heart stops.

Jiān dies.

Guan-Yin and Bohai recover.

We lose sight of them, but we begin to see the invisible traces of their sickness.

Viral particles.

Spiky infinitesimals.

On electron microscopy, they look like tiny suns, each lit with a corona of flares.

They have a name already: coronavirus.

Known, yet new, this is a novel coronavirus, SARS-CoV-2.

As yet, it is secret. Next week, all the world will know of it.

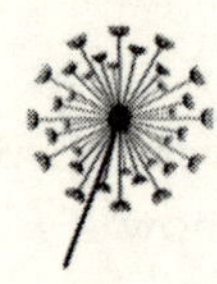

3
Landscape, Without Trees

Caesar's double-bed is warm
As an unimportant clerk
Writes I DO NOT LIKE MY WORK
On a pink official form.

– W.H. Auden, 'The Fall of Rome',
from *Nones*, 1951

COVID-19 was no surprise. After the 2003 outbreak of SARS and the 2012 outbreak of Middle East Respiratory Syndrome (MERS), it was only a matter of time before another lethal coronavirus stung us.

Why were we unprepared?

Let me rephrase that question: *Why did we let it happen again?*

We failed to prevent it because we failed to recognise a truth that stares us in the face.

It would be more correct to say we *refused* to recognise it.

Here is a litany of the landscape of this very inconvenient truth: yellow fever, zika fever, dengue, chikungunya, ebola, SARS, Nipah virus, Kyasanur Forest disease, MERS, rabies, Rocky Mountain spotted fever, sleeping sickness, hantavirus-caused diseases, Japanese encephalitis, malaria and counting …

Though these diseases are very different, their landscape of origin is the same. And it is a shockingly familiar one, no matter where you live.

It is a landscape without trees.

All these diseases emerged—or re-emerged, more virulent and dangerous—as a result of human encroachment on forests. Historically, we might trace them to tropical rainforests, but right now we must look closer to home. Because the forest was, till very recently, right here somewhere, in and about your housing colony, around that gated high-rise and its adjacent slum.

Diseases emerge when we clear forests, cut down trees, flatten hills, dam rivers, and squat on all this usurped territory.

Within a 5 km radius of my home are breeding grounds for at least seven of those listed diseases. It's not something we think about.

If we go by environmental policy alone, disease is the default position. We brag that our species achieved twelve extinctions last year, mostly insects one is duty-bound to squash. We have shoot-on-sight orders for other vermin. Our babies imbibe DDT in their very first mouthful of milk.

Can policy do more? In every way, it helps the virus push us to the brink of extinction.

Many emerging diseases, like those listed above, are zoönoses—diseases transferred from other vertebrates. Their origins can usually be traced to wildlife. They may have stayed on, unnoticed, in the wild and never made the species jump to infect us if a stable ecosystem had been left undisturbed. All our woe, with loss of Eden.

Covid-19 started this way too. Even if we haven't yet traced its origins, we've known for years that coronaviruses circulate in bats.

Bats make up 20 per cent of mammalian species. They are ubiquitous; except at the poles, they are global citizens. There is something magical about a mammal capable of sustained flight, one that can echolocate prey in the pitch-dark. Every culture, not excepting DC Comics, has substantial bat lore, and human gullibility has allowed the bat to be avidly hunted. In Southeast Asia, sixty-four species of bats are regularly exploited for meat and medicine.

The urban push into the forest forces bat populations to colonise human spaces and increases their vulnerability—and ours.

This isn't all that bad from the bat's point of view. Urbanisation provides new roosts, new sources of food and new company. Bats are sociable creatures. They form lasting relationships with home, and their urban circle of friends may embrace species that won't roost together in the wild. And this commingling means a richer, more diversified stew of bat-borne viruses.

From the virus's point of view, the bat is a bijou residence. Long lease, a little compact, yes, but comfortably air-conditioned and well connected, with a reliably frequent taxi service—can one ask for more? Apparently, a virus does.

These long-lived, vagile and generously gastronomic hosts have just one snag: bats don't get sick. Not as often as they should, considering the range of viruses they harbour. (In all, fifteen zoönotic virus families have been identified across 200 species of bats.)

Why is the bat bursting with rude health despite this terrifying arsenal of viruses?

When a bat flies, its metabolic rate rises to meet the exorbitant energy demand of flight, and its body temperature spikes to a high fever. In all mammals, fever upticks the immune process and slows viral replication. As the only mammal capable of sustained flight, the bat has evolved this pattern of spiking body temperature. The benefit is a more efficient immune system.

Bats also spend a great deal of time in torpor—a state of suspended animation, when the body's temperature drops. Was it this that encouraged viruses to co-evolve the ability to flourish across a wide range of temperatures?

Coronaviruses are 30 per cent of the healthy bat's virome. They cause diseases in other species—diarrhoeas and dysenteries; respiratory infections in cattle, dogs and swine; even peritonitis in cats. But before 2002, the worst illness they gave us humans was the common cold. Then, in 2002, SARS emerged. It had a death rate of 10 per cent. What had changed?

We know now that, before SARS erupted as epidemic, there had been small outbreaks of the disease from spillovers into civet cats and humans. A pattern was in the making.

Words like 'coincidental' and 'fortuitous' have no place in the narrative of an emerging disease. Instead, we must look for the motive force, the driver that brought about disease. Southeast Asia has lost 30 per cent of its forests in recent years. The deforested land is intensively cultivated. Urban growth is invasive. This abrupt proximity between humans and bats allows greater exposure to the viruses shed in bat saliva and guano, and provides an environment conducive to a rapidly diversifying spectrum of viruses. And since bat coronaviruses cause infections in domesticated species, intermediate hosts are aplenty.

The dynamics of the interspecies circulation of coronaviruses before they cause disease in humans are very complex, and their genomic associations are only partly known. What is known is that when there is a spillover, humans are immunologically naïve to the virus. This results in a virulent infection, and the virus quickly adapts to rapid spread between humans.

It isn't just coronaviruses that spill over from bats as we encroach on their habitat. The story of the Nipah virus is a classic of zoönosis literature. The Nipah virus first emerged in Malaysia in 1998, when Kalong bats from a deforested area roosted in a barn. Their droppings infected pigs and, eventually, the farmer. Human-to-human infection was not observed.

The Bangladesh outbreak of 2001 was a case of direct bat-to-human transmission. Date-palm (*Phoenix dactylifera*) sap is a favourite with villagers—and also with fruit-eating *Pteropus* bats. Villagers and bats shared the pot, as sap collected from the date-palm tree. This time, the virus also spread rapidly between people. This has been the pattern in both India and Bangladesh. Nipah virus is chillingly lethal—it has a mortality rate of 75 per cent.

At present, there are thousands of coronaviruses circulating in bats. Just seven of them have declared themselves in humans. As crowding increases, more may emerge. Can we predict what the next one will be like?

Absolutely not.

The West has long jeered at Asia and Africa as 'virus machines'. Such a label is deeply offensive to more than half the people on this planet, besides being scientifically untrue. Viruses are everywhere. Asia and Africa have been historically impoverished by European nations, either through genocide or colonisation. Disease was driven by conquest in the past, and racism in science is rooted in that memory. The language of science often echoes that inequality of power, and, thankfully, we're growing more sensitive to it.

Disease is driven by capitalism today: the forests of Asia, Africa, Central and South Americas are enslaved to richer nations to produce goods that serve few and bankrupt millions.

The use of forests to fuel the greed of capitalism must cease. Else, a landscape without trees may soon become a landscape without people.

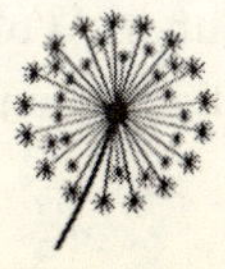

4

The Little Pin

... for within the hollow crown
That rounds the mortal temples of a king
Keeps Death his court and there the antic sits
Scoffing his state and grinning at his pomp
Allowing him a breath, a little scene,
To monarchize, be fear'd and kill with looks,
Infusing him with self and vain conceit,
As if this flesh which walls about our life
Were brass impregnable, and humor'd thus
Comes at the last, and with a little pin
Bores through his castle wall, and farewell king!

– William Shakespeare, *Richard II*

As this crown of thorns tears into our temples, Shakespeare, speaking through that weak tyrant Richard II, encapsulates the history of our species in a few lines. Our pomp and circumstance are illusions that endure in the belief that the *flesh which walls about our life were brass impregnable.*

And then we are ambushed by the unexpected:

... *thus*
Comes at the last, and with a little pin
Bores through his castle wall, and farewell king!

We have met the 'little pin' now. We have seen what it can do. But what was the build-up to this moment? The deal we had with nature when we emerged as a species—what was it?

When Covid-19 broke out in Wuhan, the news distracted me from something that had taken up the last two years.

In November 2018, I visited Dholavira, the Harappan city in Kutch, Gujarat. I returned bewildered. Between 3,000 and 1,500 BCE, Dholavira was a flourishing industrial town, probably a finishing factory on the artisanal conveyor belt. There were a number of other small towns and villages in this region which had yielded artefacts from this period. It all added up to a buzzing stone industry, which produced everything from bricks and building blocks to finely carved architectural elements and delicate jewellery.

Dholavira itself was a wonder of water conservation. Today, that is even more striking against the backdrop of the dazzling salt desert of the Rann of Kutch, but in Dholavira's heyday, the Rann was navigable sea.

Dholavira's artistic and artisanal products were exported widely and treasured as objects of value. They have been found in Babylon, in Egypt, in Oman.

And then, for no apparent reason, Dholavira had folded up.

Dholavira was perhaps one of the last Harappan towns to be abandoned. It is the relic of a complete civilisation—from inception to collapse.

Why did it collapse?

I have pondered this question for two years. It has led me to a mirror population I could examine as a model. I was neck deep in doing that, when suddenly, there was news from Wuhan.

Why do I bring this up now?

I'll answer that towards the end of this book. I mention it here because I was looking at a population that suffered very like the people of Wuhan today.

When you look at disease in the remote past, there is a living witness to what history has forgotten to record.

Archeologists and anthropologists look for human remains, thanatophiles the lot of them!

What about the living?

The human body hasn't changed, in function and design, since we emerged as *Homo sapiens sapiens* 300,000 years ago. It is to this design, and its functional response to the landscape, that we must look if we are to understand the deal we struck with the virus.

The planet had seen nothing like us before. There were stronger, bigger forms of life, and more malicious ones, but somehow we fitted in, to find our own ecological niche. Things chugged along happily till the planet hit the Holocene, 11,500 years ago. By then we had got used to being human, and had begun doing horribly human things that began to change the global environment.

Human activity dislocated natural cycles that had sustained lifeforms since they first emerged on the planet 3.8 billion years ago. As geography altered through time, it had paced the adaptation and radiation of species. Now that rhythm was disrupted by encroachment and the wilful disruption of biomes.

I suppose it all began with farming. That's the usual beginning to this narrative. But I like to push it further back, to the day we harnessed fire.

Take a quick inventory of these disruptions we've caused. They aren't termed disruptions. The usual descriptives are 'civilisation' and 'progress'. Fossil fuels have raised atmospheric carbon dioxide to levels that defy belief. Since 1750 AD, human activity has loaded the atmosphere with 555 petagrams[1] of carbon. This is likely to delay the earth's next glaciation event beyond the expected 50,000 years.

---

1. Petagram is a unit of mass equal to 10^{15} grams. Pg equals 1 billion metric tonnes.

The most ancient human profession was in practice even before we were entirely human. I know it well; it is my own, and it is 2.1 million years old.

Homo habilis, who died with his tool-kit intact, is regarded as the earliest tool-maker and user. He is usually called 'the handyman', and he was probably a surgeon. His toolkit had a knife, which he may have used to flay the prey he hunted. But he could have also used the same skills to repair, not destroy. After all, the first requirement of happy hunter-gatherers was the same as ours is today: longevity and reproduction. Injuries must heal. Babies must be delivered easily without endangering mother and child.

The use of tools evolved as much to protect and nurture as it did to weaponise the palaeo-kitchen. And tools had to be fashioned.

We discovered a quarry in every hillside. We made smart instruments. We also discovered unimaginably beautiful gems. In the Siberian Altai, the Denisova Cave has bone fragments that inaugurated a new wave of population genetics in 2010. The cave also yielded a dazzlingly beautiful artefact—a stone bracelet made of polished olivine with a high degree of finish, evidence of lapidary craft, 20,000 years ago.

Tool use—whether for butchery, for surgery, for weaponry, for making objects of great beauty, for the expression of art—inaugurated a new relationship between man and rock.

Pretty soon, we were gouging out hillsides entire.

Farming, which began around 8,000 BCE, has encroached upon forests and disrupted the rhythms of wildlife, replacing natural vegetation with cultivated strains. It has meant the relentless thinning of forests.

Consider, if you can, other life forms as people.

How many people live in a tree?

Thousands.

If you count bacteria and viruses, millions.

These displacements have meant hasty rearrangements: new homes, new sources of food, safe new nurseries, shelter from a new set of predators.

The interconnectedness of life has inspired wonder in us from the earliest times, but it has been left to poets and mystics to yammer about. The wisdom in their words has never been seen as practical advice.

It should be, now.

'Land use' is such an innocuous term for the usurpation of the earth's surface for the purpose of feeding, clothing, lodging and amusing our species. About 25–38 per cent of the net productivity is solely for human consumption—what about the rest of the species? Many have been starved, hunted and farmed to death. Quite unobtrusively, we slipped into the planet's Sixth Extinction Event.

Then came, about 500 years ago, the mass human migrations euphemistically called the 'Age of Discovery'. This period was nothing short of the genocide of two continents and the enslavement of a third. Unspeakable cruelties were perpetrated in the name of conquest and civilisation as the Americas were colonised. Over 150 years after the Spanish conquest, the population of the Americas fell from 61 million to 6 million. The 'Land of Liberty', founded on genocide, was also the agency for the largest and longest transfer of microbes across continents. The American peoples died of epidemics they had never experienced before; the Europeans took home syphilis. This was wonderfully summarised as the 'Columbian Exchange' in the 1960s.

Was syphilis unknown in Europe before 1492?

That's debatable.

What of the destruction of cultures so sophisticated that five hundred years later we survive on their skills?

Before you protest, answer this: What are the highest selling groceries during COVID-19?

Tomatoes. Potatoes. Chocolate. All gifts of the Aztecs.

Chinampas, the famed floating gardens of Tenochtitlán destroyed by Hernán Cortés, are being revived to feed a hungry Mexico reeling under COVID-19.

During this time, and for a century following, 12.5 million African men and women were captured and enslaved to work these 'New World' territories into the state of prosperity that still maintains the wealthiest nation on earth.

The British colonisation of India did not effect such genocide, but it wasn't for want of trying. Victorian India saw famines alternate with epidemics with metronomic regularity.

All pity choked with custom of fell deeds ...[2]

These are not facts that can be written without flinching, nor read without pause. Suffice it to say human cruelty is more than species betrayal: it is a declaration of war against the rest of life. The millions who die are forgotten, unnamed and unmourned, but the web of life records these wars, massacres and genocides as genetic change.

The world's geography had altered too. The ship was an intercontinental bridge for bacteria and viruses, a vector transporting disease.

---

2. *Julius Caesar*: Act 3 Scene 1.
Mark Anthony ends this segment with:
Cry 'Havoc!' and let slip the dogs of war,
That this foul deed shall smell above the earth
With carrion men, groaning for burial.

Look now at the last hundred years. With the introduction of industrial conversion of atmospheric nitrogen into ammonia for fertiliser, the nitrogen cycle was breached. This is a very deep injury to the planet's stability. All life forms are in a mad scramble to reset this imbalance—and this usually means a genetic change for advantage under these new conditions. The last time something this drastic happened was 2.5 million years ago.

After 1950, human activity has been in a sustained overdrive.

A new high in human destructiveness was achieved with the atomic explosions of 1945. All nations should have instinctively sworn 'Never Again'.

But we didn't, did we?

We left a permanent signature of violence in the air. The C_{14} level has been used as a marker since 1963; we talk glibly of 'carbon dating', and we overlook that it is a marker of our callousness and brutality towards our own.

What has human activity done to the non-human population of the planet? Animal extinctions, plant extinctions—these we do notice. What we don't notice are the pixels of loss that add up to extinction.

Sometimes, those missing pixels alter only a very circumscribed territory—say the vegetation at our doorstep. I witnessed this last year, when the annual municipal pre-monsoon tree-trimming turned into an orgy of mindless brutality, our protesting voices drowned in the whine of electric chainsaws.

I was asked righteously: 'Haven't you read how many people are killed by falling trees? Better safe than sorry. Trees will grow again, but can you restore a human life?'

Before such bathos, indignation subsides to a grumble.

Nobody asked the vital question: *How many people live on a tree?*

The tree canopy (defined as the part of a plant above ground, not just the aerial canopies of tall trees) is home to 30 million species—and counting. When my trees stood tall and brave, I knew some of their inhabitants by appearance, others by song and chatter, still more by the traces they left of a hedonic lifestyle—badam fruit bleeding on the ground, a half-eaten mango, red-violet spatters of yesterday's gluttony on the jamun tree. Others I identified for their nuisance value of buzz, crawl, sting and whirr.

With typical human arrogance, I had simply negated other, less visible life-forms.

To ecologists today, the tree canopy is an undiscovered continent—and exploring it is difficult, hazardous and sometimes practically impossible. The pioneers in this challenging field, Nalini Nadkarni and Margaret Lowman, have brought to light amazing facts about the tops of trees. Treetops are autonomous, their machinery of life working independently of the forest floor. Their insect and animal populations thrive interdependently.

All these populations had been evicted by the mindless felling of a small ring of trees. Where would they go?

Unfortunately, I know the answer.

Through 2016, as I followed the Zika pandemic, incident by incident, what ought to have been a glaring fact stayed a well-kept secret. It is worthwhile to remind ourselves of the timeline. In the Zika forest of Uganda, the virus was isolated from a test rhesus monkey kept chained on a high platform, level with the tree's canopy. The year was 1947.

The mosquito that bit the monkey lived up there.

At that time, the Zika virus was responsible for the occasional flu-like illness that humans who lived around the forest sometimes reported. Those trees were felled. Human habitation increased. The forest was thinned out.

The mosquito vector *Aedes aegypti* is identified as a night-biting, tree-hole dweller. *Äedes aegypti* adapted smartly, and swiftly, to a modern convenience as nursery for its eggs—water containers. It now wings about at a much lower level and has switched its feeding schedule to human hours, biting by day.

Fifty years is a long time, and all this while, Zika fever appeared sporadically as just that—a mild fever, with no outfall. And then came its Brazilian iteration in 2015. The horrific new manifestation caused foetal disruption across the placenta, resulting in the birth of microcephalic babies, with damaged brains and eyes. All research and comment that followed ignored just one truth. Deforestation.

Almost the entire planet is now a refugee camp for mosquitoes that once lived safe in tree canopies. The viruses they carry are no longer innocent bystanders. They have emerged as killer pathogens.

And they move into my home—or yours—each time we cut down a tree.

We have broken the covenant of coexistence in so many ways and for so long, it is shocking we noticed the consequences only recently.

The little pin that brings about disaster isn't always evident. It isn't even a century since we became aware of how to look for it when a disease emerges.

Cause and effect, though, have been noticed in every age, by every culture. A tenth-century Kannada mystic Dasareswara sang:

Knowing one's lowliness in every word;
the scatter of insects in the air in every gesture of the hand;
things living, things moving, come sprung from the earth under every footfall;
and when holding a plant or joining it to another or in the letting it go
to be all mercy
to be light
as a dusting brush of peacock feathers:
such moving, such awareness
is love that makes us one
with the Lord, Dasareswara!

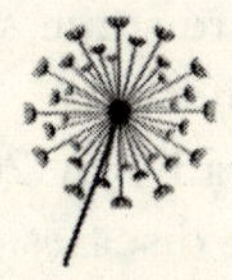

5

7.8 Billion Sitting Ducks

I should have stayed at home
'Cause I was doing better alone.

– Dua Lipa, 'Break My Heart',
from *Future Nostalgia*, 2020

More people die of conditions other than COVID-19 all through the year. Here are some statements that appear, at first glance, to be unconnected:

~ Of 56 million deaths in 2017, 73.4 per cent were from non-communicable diseases. The three leading causes of these deaths were cardiovascular diseases, cancers and diabetes.

Among the 21 per cent who died of communicable diseases, a very large percentage died of lower respiratory tract infections.

~ In 2016, more than 1.9 billion adults were overweight. Of these, over 650 million were obese.

Among Asians, the connection between obesity and cardiovascular illness is more pronounced. Both China and India are facing epidemics of obesity.

~ As of 2019, 463 million adults have diagnosed diabetes. In 2000, the number was 151 million.

There were 4.3 million deaths from diabetes in 2019.

In 2016, the number of diabetics in India was estimated at 65 million. The disease was most prevalent in Tamil Nadu and Kerala, followed by Punjab and Goa.

China has the highest number of diabetics in the world.

~ Lower respiratory tract infections kill more than 4 million people every year.

Respiratory diseases make up 5 per cent of the commonest causes of death.

~ In India, 1.24 million deaths were attributed to air pollution, including 0.67 million to particulate matter air pollution and 0.48 million to household air pollution.

India's Air Quality Index (AQI) is dangerously high.

~ Particulate matter air pollution is identified as one of the highest health risks in China.

These six facts, which appear so random, have a common denominator. They are connected by a similarity in the body's response: these illnesses damage body organs and alter systemic processes through the response of inflammation.

While inflammation is a highly conserved protective response, it can go drastically wrong. In non-communicable diseases—like obesity, diabetes and heart disease—not only is inflammation seriously disordered, it can also precipitate life-threatening emergencies.

These diseases present chronic inflammatory states. Different though they may appear, they do have a common disorder in cellular function. To understand this better, forget for a moment various diagnostic labels like heart disease, obesity or diabetes. Just think of a state in which you feel unwell without being actually sick.

Most of us have experienced that.

We have words to convey that spectrum of discomfort. Yours may not be mine, but the feeling is all too familiar.

Sadly, too many people suffer from these discomfiting feelings most of the time. Too many people wheeze and cough as a matter of course, are overweight, hypertensive, diabetic, arthritic. Too many people are chronically ill but don't have the time, or else think it self-indulgent, to notice it.

Too many people have chronic inflammation.

Think of this as a grumbling state of cellular backchat, where the body is sassing the usual regulatory mechanisms. When inflammation slips the leash and goes rogue, it is silly season for complications. A virus, which could have been batted off easily by the immune system, now gets house room. This happens because rogue inflammation makes many immune processes shut down. Very quickly, the body is infected.

That's just the beginning of the story, surely?

Things can fall back in order, can't they?

What about adaptive immunity, the learnt response of hitting back at infection? Can inflammation cripple that too?

Not only can it do that, it can go on to achieve worse. It can overturn most protective responses into actively destructive ones, making the body practically fall in with the virus's agenda. And so the infection becomes life-threatening.

As can happen with Covid-19.

Will that happen to the 7.8 billion of us?

For we are a population primed for disaster, existing, no matter where we belong, in a state of low-grade chronic inflammation induced by our way of life.

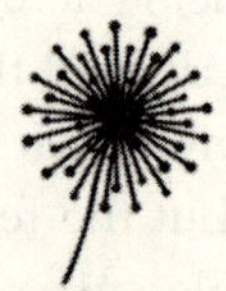

6
Disease

> Nothing matches the holiness and fascination
> of accurate and intricate detail.
>
> – Stephen Jay Gould, *I Have Landed*, 2002

Disease is a word we use thoughtlessly because of the meaning it's had for centuries: *illness.*

Look closer at the word, and it reveals the unexpected.

Have you ever accidentally shelled a wormy pea-pod? Think of that moment when you opened the pod. In that split second before you chucked the pod with a shudder, remember what you saw? Movement. Destruction. Spoilage. Debris.

And in the midst of all that chaos, you might have just about noticed the worm within. You might have registered the textured colour-scape. A pea-pod is a statement of green—satin smooth, opaque. But that glimpse would have revealed something more elemental, ochre and grey ore, crumbled between sand and paste, carrying but a semblance of green.

Disease is that disruption of form and substance, that confusion of spirit and dislodgment of purpose.

Nobody confuses disease with unease. 'I feel uneasy' is very different from 'I have a disease'. The first is perception, the second—information. Yet, both words are rooted in 'ease', which is our expected state of existence, the state we should call *usual* but generally describe as *normal.*

Unease is the perception of disturbance.

Disease is ease corrupted and unrecognisable, transformed into a mask of suffering.

Disease is chaos.

The original Greek idea of chaos actually described the opposite. Chaos was the state of *being*. This is a very modern thought in the time of Covid-19, when disease seems to have become our state of being,

When we look at the chaos that is Covid-19, it is like that glimpse into a wormy pea-pod. The language of Covid-19 is full of panic: emergence, spread, pandemic. Or despair: distancing, isolation, quarantine, lockdown, curfew, desolation, death.

But consider the still point.

This moment, when you and I are conversing on this page, exchanging thought. Strangers, yet intimate in our quest for reason, order, indeed, life—a return to ease.

This moment, this scintilla of human existence, encapsulates the totality of human experience—intelligence, perception, thought. The perfect counterpoise to panic and despair.

So let's take a logical look at disease.

Disease is a quarrel within the body.

An external element may start off the quarrel, or 'incite the disturbance', as a newspaper might put it. But the quarrel is within the body, among its own family members, many of whom reveal unexpected facets and behave in unimaginable ways.

Medical science is focused on understanding these facets as they reveal themselves, and then imagining and anticipating their consequences so that they don't recur. Sadly, much of medicine is hindsight. But hindsight can become recall that is timely and analytical.

Science is all about thinking on your feet when up to your eyebrows in a mess like Covid-19. Okay, up to your neck.

We think of a disease like COVID-19 as an infection—the invasion of the body by a harmful outside element—but that is the lesser half of the story.

Infection is the unhappy ending.

Immunity is the happy ending.

Like all great stories, COVID-19 is a tragedy, a love story gone seriously wrong.

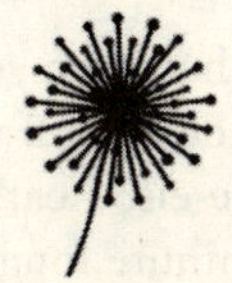

7
What is a Virus?

The past and present wilt—I have fill'd them,
emptied them.
And proceed to fill my next fold of the future.

Listener up there! what have you to confide to me?
Look in my face while I snuff the sidle of evening,
(Talk honestly, no one else hears you, and I stay only
a minute longer.)

Do I contradict myself?
Very well then I contradict myself,
(I am large, I contain multitudes.)

I concentrate toward them that are nigh, I wait on
the door-slab.

Who has done his day's work? who will soonest be
through with his supper?
Who wishes to walk with me?

Will you speak before I am gone? will you prove
already too late?

– Walt Whitman, *Song of Myself*, Section 51, 1855

By now every kindergartener knows what the coronavirus looks like. Older children can identify that spiky ball as an RNA virus. The press might enlarge on this, but only slightly. A research paper on the internet might announce breathlessly: *The coronavirus is an enveloped, non-segmented, positive-sense RNA virus.*

But what do all these words mean?

How do they equip us to face the crisis of COVID-19?

The language of social media has shortened attention spans to 140 bytes, just long enough to grab at a thought before it whizzes past.

If we slow down and look closer at what the words mean, they will inform and elucidate.

The quickest way to understand a word is to question it.

What is a virus?

Something invisible that causes a dangerous illness?

Yes—invisible to the naked eye because it is infinitesimal, but visible at great magnification under an electron microscope (EM). And yes, it is often a dangerous illness that declares the presence of a virus.

This makes up the narrative of discovery.

The dangerous illness that led to the discovery of viruses did not affect humans. The victims were tobacco plants in Holland. They withered from a sudden blight and crippled a very lucrative industry. Naturally, this was seen as a crisis—anything that endangers money always is—and the best brains were put to work to produce a solution.

Over the next few years, scientists discovered facts that explain a lot about our present crisis. The extract from infected plants could rapidly infect healthy plants on contact. When this extract was passed through a filter whose pores were too small to admit bacteria, the filtrate was still infectious. Clearly, the infection was caused by an organism or substance even smaller than bacteria.

Martinus Willem Beijerinck of Delft looked still further. The year was 1898. He found that, although the entire plant was infectious, the heaviest load of infection came from young leaves. Beijerlink concluded that the infecting organism was not capable of independent existence but reached its peak within the rapidly dividing cells of young leaves. This was a brilliant insight. Beijerlink called this infectious agent *contagium vivum fluidum*, or contagious living fluid, and later, he changed it to the much snappier 'virus'. Today, Beijerinck's subject is called the tobacco mosaic virus.

Virus, a word so familiar to us today, has its ancient roots in the Sanskrit word 'visham', or poison. 'Vish' described the quality of being pervasive. It was in this sense that it entered Latin in the fourteenth century, when it was used to describe sticky plant sap—echoed in the English word 'viscid'. In the 1700s, 'virus' was used to characterise the 'new' malady of syphilis. After Beijerinck used the word to describe a highly infective organism, virus found its niche in the dictionary.

Though the term was in common use in the early years of the twentieth century, nobody had seen a virus yet. The question 'what is a virus?' was still unanswered.

Then, in 1931, Ernst Ruska and Max Knoll built the first EM. In 1939, the first virus Ruska and his colleagues took a good close look at was Beijerinck's tobacco mosaic virus. New viruses were discovered using electron microscopy. In 1948, the EM revealed the difference between the viruses that cause smallpox and chicken pox. In 1952, the poliovirus showed up. Practically every year since, we've been gathering facts on virus structure and appearance.

We've been staring at viruses for a century now, so what *are* they?

They're incessantly described as particles, as in viral particles. Sounds pejorative, if you ask me; the virus is a life form, isn't it? *Is* it?

The jury's still out on that, believe it or not, so let's sift the evidence.

A virus is a jot of nucleic acid in a protein jacket. The nucleic acid, either RNA or DNA, is the virus's persona, its genome. The jacket is protection against hostile elements.

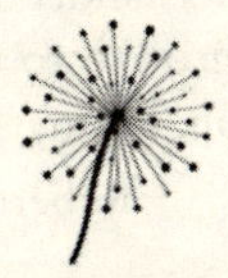

8

Our Sixty Years With Coronavirus

We have short time to stay, as you,
We have as short a spring;
As quick a growth to meet decay,
As you, or anything.

– Robert Herrick, 'To Daffodils', 1665

Finding a cure for the common cold is a joke so hoary, it is a meme.

The common cold sparked the discovery of coronaviruses. We have known coronaviruses for sixty years. That is a long time in science—a time of feverish question and discovery.

In 1965, David A.J. Tyrrell and M.L. Bynoe reported a new virus, and they named it B-814. They discovered its presence in cells cultured from the respiratory tract of an adult with a severe cold. Meanwhile, two other researchers, Dorothy Hamre and John Procknow, had grown another virus, also in cultures obtained from what must have been a very curious lot of volunteers—medical students with colds. I can imagine how they must have jostled for a look at their contributions to history. Hamre and Procknow called their virus 229-E.

B-814 and 229-E, and a virus that caused respiratory disease in chickens, all looked alike. Medium-sized (80–150 nm), on EM, their most striking feature was a crown of club- or petal-shaped surface projections—'peplomers' or 'spikes'. And that crown-like, dazzling surface armour decided the name of this newly discovered family of viruses: Coronaviridae or 'crowned viruses'.

Coronaviruses, as we now know them, have a fatty envelope and a single strand of RNA as genome. It was soon found that they weren't restricted to humans and chickens. The lexicon of lurgy swelled: swine gastroenteritis, mouse hepatitis, human colds and bronchitis, respiratory diseases in birds, peritonitis in cats …

The clinical information about coronaviruses over the next few decades was sparse. They were found in secretions from common colds and caused respiratory illnesses, but were not considered particularly dangerous. Most infections were upper respiratory, with the occasional pneumonia in children and bronchitis in the elderly.

We learnt more about the structure and distribution of coronaviruses. They seemed to infect a very wide spectrum of species and cause a variety of illnesses. Rodents, swine, felines, canines, birds, bovines—the count grew. And the diseases? Coronaviruses could target every body system, it seemed!

The coronavirus genome and its synthesis of proteins was studied. Coronaviruses were found to have a very high recombination rate. In recombination, viruses of two different parent strains co-infect the same host cell and interact during replication to generate virus progeny that have genes from both parents—a marriage of true viral minds. This high recombination rate explained the wide host spectrum of coronaviruses, and their ability to evolve into more pathogenic forms.

The crowning glory of coronaviruses, the spike, was revealed to have two active component parts that must be split before the virus can infect the host cell. Spike protein cleavage depended upon the strain of the virus and the type of host cell.

In 1987, the first genomic sequencing of a coronavirus was accomplished on the infectious bronchitis (IB) virus. And then, in 2002, came SARS, a killer coronavirus infection. The virus isolated in this outbreak could be grown quickly in cultures, and that led to early genomic sequencing. The infecting virus was not a known human coronavirus, but a novel pathogen, closely related to a coronavirus known to infect the masked palm civet. The meat of palm civets is considered a delicacy in China and Vietnam, and the animal is regular merchandise.

Palm civet coronavirus has a 29-nucleotide sequence, absent in viruses collected from human victims of SARS. It seemed that knocking this sequence out had made the species jump possible. A large number of vendors in the wet markets of Gangzhou who sold and handled palm civets were seropositive for the SARS virus—without having suffered any symptoms at all. This meant the virus had been circulating long enough for this population to have developed adaptive immunity against it: an observation of great relevance in this, our present, pandemic.

The palm civet coronavirus was subsequently traced to a bat coronavirus. Horseshoe bats are today regarded as reservoir hosts for the SARS virus.

In 2012, MERS emerged. This infection passed from camel to human, camels having acquired it from bats. It had a much higher case mortality than SARS, 38 per cent.

Both SARS and MERS-CoV were respiratory illnesses; pneumonias that could lead to the frightening acute respiratory distress syndrome (ARDS).

With this information, we expected other, novel coronaviruses to emerge as fresh zoönoses that again would have dire effects on the respiratory system. We didn't have to wait very long, did we?

SARS-CoV-2 emerged in Wuhan in November 2019. It leads to the pneumonia we call COVID-19. The fatal complication is the same as that in SARS and MERS-CoV.

In fact, the same complication kills in a lot of other diseases as well.

Which is why I feel this pandemic demands a closer look at ARDS.

And ARDS is *not* caused by the virus.

It is caused by us.

The deciding factor of the outcome in COVID-19 is not SARS-CoV-2.

It is our response to it.

It is what happens within the lungs.

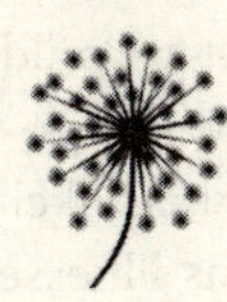

9
Before December 2019

A good traveller has no fixed plan and is not intent on arriving.

– Lao Tzu

The coronavirus family is huge, so for convenience, coronaviruses are grouped as alpha coronaviruses, beta coronaviruses, delta coronaviruses and gamma coronaviruses.

Their host range is wide. Coronaviruses cause any number of illnesses in birds and mammals. Some of these are killer diseases, but most are mild and soon forgotten. The farming industry should be our go-to space for information about coronaviruses and their likely reservoirs.

In humans, coronavirus illnesses involve the respiratory tract. They may also infect in other ways, but we've become most familiar with commonplace illnesses, like a bad cold, and with killer diseases like SARS and MERS.

What did we know before December 2019 that could have warned us of the coming plague?

We knew of the coronavirus's potential to infect quickly and fatally.

We knew its wildlife reservoir.

We also knew that the coronavirus is quick to make the species jump and emerge as a dangerous illness with rapid human-to-human infection.

In 2003, there were 8,096 cases and 774 deaths from SARS. It was very nearly a pandemic. The fatality rate was 9.6 per cent

MERS-CoV is still grumbling somewhere, considering that between April 2012 and October 2018, there were 2,229 laboratory-confirmed cases reported globally. Of these people, 791 died. That's a frighteningly high figure. It works out to a fatality rate of 35.5 per cent.

In reality, numbers carry no meaning. They don't answer the questions: *Are my loved ones safe? Am I?*

The second question is even more important than the first. To care for your loved ones, you have to be well.

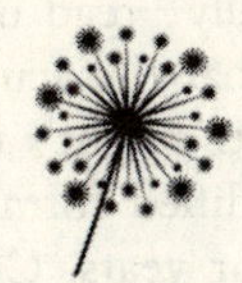

10
Naming the Beast

I remember going to the British Museum one day to read up the treatment for some slight ailment of which I had a touch—hay fever, I fancy it was. I got down the book, and read all I came to read; and then, in an unthinking moment, I idly turned the leaves, and began to indolently study diseases, generally ... and so started alphabetically—read up ague, and learnt that I was sickening for it, and that the acute stage would commence in about another fortnight. Bright's disease, I was relieved to find, I had only in a modified form, and, so far as that was concerned, I might live for years. Cholera I had, with severe complications; and diphtheria I seemed to have been born with. I plodded conscientiously through the twenty-six letters, and the only malady I could conclude I had not got was housemaid's knee.

–Jerome K. Jerome, *Three Men In a Boat (To Say Nothing of the Dog)*, 1889

This classic description of the Google specialist at work was written a century before the internet. The only malady the author limped home without—housemaid's knee—would not be a politically correct ailment today. He would have to splutter his way past pre-patellar bursitis, as we splutter over his name, Jerome Klapka Jerome.

Richard Bright was a London physician who spent most of his life documenting kidney diseases. Honours came thick and fast, but he hadn't actually arrived till a disease was named after him. It was the physician's pinnacle of glory, and an overcrowded one, even in Bright's time. Were Bright alive today, he would have to be content with a Nobel, letting his disease go as nephritis.

People can no longer be diseases (Addison's disease, Bright's disease, Crohn's disease, Hodgkin's lymphoma, Klinefelter's syndrome, Salmonellosis, Tay-Sachs disease).

Nor can places (German measles, Spanish flu, Lassa fever, Guinea worm, Ross River fever, La Crosse encephalitis, Lyme disease).

Nor can professions—the Mad Hatter would be trolled by infuriated fashionistas.

Nor can other species (monkeypox, avian influenza).

There is reason enough for these precautions while naming a disease: the past is full of misunderstandings, prejudice, misogyny and racism. So is the healthy present—but we can, at least, avoid them while naming ailments.

The classic case of a misnomer is syphilis. Its first mention comes two years after Columbus's historic voyage to Guanahani, which resulted in the 'discovery of America' and the genocide of Native Americans. The first to be affected by the disease were Neapolitan sailors, but Italy was then being overrun by the French, so the first to be identified as infected with this new plague was a French soldier. Italians called it the French disease. The French, of course, called it the Italian, sometimes the Neapolitan, disease. Syphilis border-hopped across Europe over the next fifty years, always being blamed on the enemy of the day. It was in turn French, Italian, Russian and Polish, until Girolamo Fracastoro, the polymath of Padua, took charge of the disease in a poem whose central character, the shepherd boy Syphilus, contracts the disease. It reads vile in English and is hopefully better in the original Italian:

He first wore Buboes dreadful to the sight,
First felt strange pains and sleepless past the Night;
From him the Malady receiv'd its name,
The neighbouring Shepherds catch'd the spreading Flame.

Fracastoro was lucky. With his poem,[3] he managed to escape all of the World Health Organisation's (WHO's) provisos, and syphilis will stay syphilis till the end of time. Mediocrity wins, every time.

When syphilis arrived in India, it was part of the Portuguese gift package of tomatoes, potatoes, rubber and cashews. Naturally, it was called 'firangi rog', the white man's disease.

In recent times, we have had misnomers like the Spanish flu. The influenza pandemic of 1918—that killed over 50 million worldwide—began early the morning of 4 March, when Private Albert Gitchell of the US Army reported sick at Fort Riley, in the Flint Hills of Kansas. By afternoon, 100 more had fallen ill.

The Marburg virus emerged in miners working near a cave in Uganda, but was named for the town in Germany where the virus was isolated.

SARS-CoV-2 is responsible for the fifth zoönosis out of China in the recent past. China has suffered racism and Chinese people have been stigmatised shamefully since this epidemic broke. The virus was initially dubbed the Wuhan virus, then the 'novel coronavirus-2019', and then the 'Covid-19 virus'. It wasn't until 12 February that the WHO announced official names for both virus and disease.

SARS-CoV-2, the name given to the virus, is logical enough as an addendum to the earlier SARS outbreak, also caused by a coronavirus. The name was decided on by the Coronavirus Study Group of the International Committee on the Taxonomy of Viruses. An RNA virus, the SARS-CoV-2 has a high mutation rate. Like all RNA viruses, it

---

3. *Syphilis Sive Morbus Gallicus* (Syphilis or The French Disease), 1530.

has a gene called RNA-dependent RNA polymerase, *RdRp;* if two RNA viruses need to be compared with each other, this is the gene to check out. The Coronavirus Study Group found that the *RdRp* genes of this newly emerged virus and that causing SARS were similar. They concluded this new virus and SARS-CoV were closely related and so named it SARS-CoV-2.

The WHO accepted this unhappily. It feared people would panic at the recall of SARS, especially in Asia. The WHO still refers to it 'the virus that causes COVID-19'.

Predictably, every country will use the tag closest to its own language. India adopted 'corona' early, dropped the 'virus' and flexed its muscles on: Go, Corona, Go! The term is never pronounced corona, but karona, which breaks up nicely into karo-na, in the north. Nobody has thought of calling it 'karuna virus', which is a pity as the subcontinent could certainly use a booster of karuna, compassion, right now.

COVID-19, the name given to the disease, is just telegraph for corona virus disease of 2019. It is terse, easily pronounced and completely inoffensive, even if it sounds more like a detergent than a dangerous disease.

COVID-19 can be explained thus:

Category: Coronavirus
Realm: Riboviria
Order: Nidovirales
Suborder: Comidovirinae
Family: Coronaviridae
Subfamily: Orthocoronavirinae
Genus: Betacoronovirus
Subgenus: Sarbecoronavirus
Species: Severe Respiratory Syndrome Related Coronavirus

Individuum: SARS-CoVUrbani, SARS-CoVGZ-02, Bat SARS CoVRf1/2004,

Civet SARSCoVSZ3/2003, SARS-CoVPC4-227, SARSr-CoVBtKY72,

SARS-CoV-2 Wuhan-Hu-1, SARSr-CoVRatG13, and so on.

To me, COVID resonates with Ovid, the Roman poet, author of *Metamorphosis*, a book dedicated to the change of form induced by circumstance. The *Metamorphosis* is about a passel of unfortunate mortals forced to flee their bodies and inhabit others to escape persecution from assorted gods and goddesses. It could just as well be a primer of virology: protean, unpredictable, legion in its manifestations.

Let Ovid recount a simpler story:

Of bodies chang'd to various forms, I sing:
Ye Gods, from whom these miracles did spring,
Inspire my numbers with coelestial heat;
'Till I my long laborious work compleat:
And add perpetual tenour to my rhimes,
Deduc'd from Nature's birth, to Caesar's times.

Like all viruses, the SARS-CoV-2 has evolved through this pandemic to produce different clades. These may manifest as different clinical profiles, but not necessarily more dangerous ones. SARS-CoV-2's mutation rate assures a slightly different genome with every replication. Such a viral population, with a number of different genomes, is called a quasispecies. Ovid would have recognised the phenomenon as … metamorphosis.

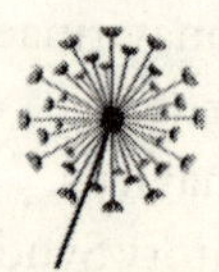

11
The Battle Within the Cell

After such knowledge, what forgiveness?

– T. S. Eliot, 'Gerontion',
from *Poems*, 1920

The cell is a walled maze. The wall is a very complicated ID checkpoint. It is guarded by receptors. These molecules are gossips: sometimes credulous, sometimes canny. And at some other times, as in the case of a viral infection, simply asking for trouble by collaborating with the enemy.

When a receptor binds with a molecule, signals are set off. 'Signalling' involves a temporary chemical change in the molecule. It can revert to its original state when the job is done.

In addition to these big molecules that cut such a swagger, there are lowly molecules that carry out humbler functions towards the same end. These are desultorily called 'second messengers', but their importance shouldn't be overlooked.

Once a virus enters the cell it must navigate the intracellular maze. Here, it will encounter many cellular pathways. In cell biology, a pathway is a little different from the familiar pagdandi. A pathway is a set of reactions by which cellular enzymes transform a molecule to make it perform or influence a function.

The virus has to zigzag its way through several such intersecting pathways to achieve its goal of replication. In the process, it cripples and destroys the machinery of the host cell. By the time the second generation makes its exit, the cell will have changed in a number of ways as a result of the virus-host interaction.

These are some important pathways along which virus and host interact:

> Autophagy, literally eating oneself, is an ancient trick all body cells possess. Autophagy is a response to cell stress (which is not your usual Monday morning). One of the commonest forms of cell stress is starvation—even a day's fasting qualifies. In response to stress, cell organelles are sequestered, packaged and digested. Deprived of its machinery, the cell weakens functionally and structurally. In a state of health, autophagy is often protective to the host. When under attack, the autophagy pathway makes the cell vulnerable to rapid destruction. Coronaviruses like SARS-CoV-2 take over important molecules in this pathway and divert them for their own benefit to increase replication.

> Apoptosis,[4] or programmed cell death. This is a means of genetic control. When apoptosis is activated, the cell is dismantled. Imagine dismantling your house, taking down wall cupboards, moving furniture, turning up mattresses—and then think of this happening within the cell.

All body processes are neat and economical, even programmed cell death: the cell organelles are bundled up into a neat packed lunch for the next wandering phagocyte,[5] and the cell dies. Phagocytes are white blood cells whose job it is to swallow particles identified as either dangerous

---

4. From Greek *apo* = separation + *ptosis* = falling off.

5. Phagocytes are cells that protect organisms by engulfing infecting agents, foreign bodies and dead matter. They are the first echelon of defense and also of immunity. They were discovered by the Russian zoologist Élie Metchnikoff in 1882. He would share the Nobel Prize in 1908 with the German physician Paul Ehrlich for the explication of immunity. Phagocyte combines the Greek *phagein*, 'to eat', with *kutos*, 'hollow vessel', which gives us the word cell.

Schoolchildren know, from their first lessons in biology, about how the unicellular amoeba eats, moves and fights by employing phagocytosis. It means that this phenomenon arose very early in the evolution of life.

The white blood cells are the professional phagocytes that circulate in human blood.

or messy. So when a phagocyte arrives near a cell that has undergone apoptosis, it grabs a quick lunch, mops the counter clean and sails away.

Because apoptosis is genetically programmed, it does not incite the immune response. It is a quiet, 'normal' body event.

But coronaviruses like SARS-CoV-2 disinhibit apoptosis. Because SARS-CoV-2 is an inhaled virus, apoptosis begins in the cells lining the airway. In addition, cells of the blood vessel lining, the nervous system, the spleen, the liver, lymphocytes and more … are all pushed into apoptosis by the virus. Imagine the damage! It is uncontrolled, uncontrollable, cell death.

> Endoplasmic reticulum (ER) stress response is another important cellular pathway that is hijacked by the virus. The ER is the cell organelle where synthesised proteins are folded and modified. Under stress, the amounts of protein synthesised and folded can vary. If the ER is full, unfolded proteins pile up and produce ER stress. A coronavirus infection sets this off dramatically by upping the protein load on the ER. This leads to a response called the unfolded protein response, which results in massive cell death through apoptosis.

The host fights viral invasion through immunity. The first response, the one to an unknown pathogen, is innate immunity. Innate immunity depends on the host's immune cells. Viruses can subvert the host's immune cells directly, or sneakily get the host itself to do so.

Clearly, this has been going on for millions of years, long before we were mammals—or the pathways of immunity would not be so firmly entrenched in us, nor so cleverly outwitted by the virus.

This is how a mere jot of RNA can successfully hijack stable and functional cellular pathways for its own use. The body's defences are not merely countered but utterly subverted by the virus. This coup d'état achieves the virus's simple agenda of infinite replication.

The result on the host is not so simple.

Viral infection results in the destruction and death of the individual cell, through the processes we glimpsed in this chapter.

But the 'individual cell' isn't what we notice, is it?

What is the noticeable result of this battle within the cell?

In different species, coronaviruses attack different tissues, giving rise to a wide spectrum of illnesses.

The coronavirus that causes COVID-19 attacks the respiratory tract.

What makes the human respiratory tract such a haven for coronaviruses?

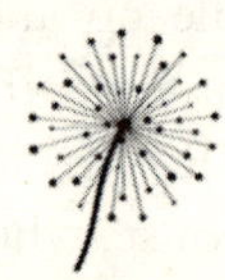

12

The Airway

What happens to a dream deferred?
Does it dry up
like a raisin in the sun?
– Langston Hughes, 'Harlem',
from *Montage of a Dream Deferred*, 1951

I like to use the term airway for the respiratory system, because it encapsulates function and anatomy neatly.

The visible parts of the airway are economical: the nose, specifically the nostrils and nasal cavity, and the mouth. The concealed spread is much more lavish.

Behind the features recognisable as your face is the upper extension of the airway—a labyrinth of spaces tunnelled through the bones of the forehead and the cheeks, extending to the ear on either side. A further extension is located behind the top of the nose and is roofed by the most exalted part of the body—the brain. These tunnels are the sinuses. And because they are contiguous to the nasal cavities, they are called paranasal sinuses. Sinuses are air pockets with delicate and sensitive linings. They are likely to be more important than we have realised in coronavirus infections.[6]

The lower airway, which leads off from the throat, is guarded by a leaf-like structure called the epiglottis. This

6. The reason should have been perfectly obvious from the start to anyone with a working knowledge of Covid-19, but the pundits are only waking up to it months into the pandemic. Let us spare their blushes, and save it for the end of this book.

saves your life by preventing you from choking when you swallow too hastily. Anything that comes into contact with the epiglottis makes you cough. Remember, *cough is protective.*

This lower respiratory tract that the epiglottis guards begins with the trachea. This is the rigid tube you can feel in the midline in the front of your neck. You lose sight of it beyond your collarbones because, at this point, it dives into the chest cavity. At about the level of the breastbone, the trachea bifurcates into bronchi. Each bronchus now branches like a tree. Think of the twigs on a tree as bronchioles; like twigs, bronchioles become softer and more elastic the further they are from the parent branch. Each bronchiole ends in a tiny elastic bag nested in a mesh of fine blood vessels—this is the alveolus. The alveoli, together with the scaffolding of bronchioles and blood vessels, make up the right and left lungs.

We need both our lungs in working order to breathe effectively.

Each lung has a thin, lubricated, double-layered covering, the pleura. In health, the two layers of pleura are in close contact. In diseased states, they may become separated by clear or infected fluid. As a result, the lungs will have less space for expansion.

Think of the airway as a tube with a teabag at one end, dangled into the bloodstream. Clean air goes in, and oxygen is exchanged for carbon dioxide through the teabag. Then, dirty with carbon dioxide, air must rush back out again. Described thus, it seems a complicated manoeuvre. But it is so easy we are seldom aware that we are breathing—till we fall sick. The airway is a very complicated place to get sick in, full of challenges and short on resource.

The work of breathing is kept smooth and unnoticeable by muscles. The ones we do notice are between the ribs and beneath it—the intercostal muscles and the diaphragm. These muscles make the chest wall move. They act like bellows to fill and empty the lungs with air. There are other muscles we only notice when it becomes difficult to breathe. These are the muscles of the face and neck, which then begin to strain under the effort of breathing.

The bigger tubes of the airway have bits of cartilage in their walls to stent them and keep them from collapsing. As the airway branches to smaller than 2 mm units, cartilage disappears.

The last part of the airway is the alveolus, the terminal elastic 'teabag' that does the actual work of breathing—gas exchange. There are two special kinds of cells here.

One is responsible for gas exchange. The other secretes a molecule called surfactant, which keeps the alveolus from collapsing.

Breathing *is* gas exchange.

The point of respiration is to ensure adequate oxygen with every breath and to throw out carbon dioxide. So, no matter which part of the airway flubs on the job, and no matter how, things get dangerous when gas exchange is threatened.

In Covid-19, as illness worsens, gas exchange is impaired. Death occurs when oxygenation can no longer be sustained.

The airway is far from being a passive tube. It is intrinsic to the body's first line of defence.

There are many types of airway cells: basal cells, ciliated cells, mucus-producing goblet cells, club cells and neuroendocrine cells. In this discussion, we'll consider them all, simply, as airway cells.

Airway cells form a continuum of integrity, a reliable defence layer between the inhaled air and the more delicate population of the cells deeper in the airway. This barrier relies on a biological entity—the luminal junctional complex—which acts as a glue between cells, to toughen it. When weakened, the lining becomes prone to attack by invading microbes or inhaled particles like pollutants and allergens. Long-standing or intermittent breathing problems like asthma—as well as sudden respiratory infections—begin with a failure of this first defensive layer.

Defence is one thing, but the airway also has a fail-safe population of cells for repair. These stem cells can generate new, specialised cells to restore tissue wear and tear.

The airway, like other parts of the body, has its own resident population of 'good' microbes—the lung microbiome. Changes in the lung microbiome can mean the difference between health and respiratory disease.

But all these defence systems are useless without information.

How does the airway lining get its smarts about inhaled air?

The airway cell has its own intelligence network. Harmful molecules are recognised when they come into contact with receptors on the cell surface or within.

What is harmful?

Anything that is recognised as non-self. This can include particulate matter, bacteria, fungi—and, of course, viruses.

The intelligence network centralises its information in a posse of response molecules. These set off chemical reactions which produce effector molecules to switch on the process of defence we call immunity.

Immunity is big, messy, operatic. It plays out on an overcrowded stage. The temperamental characters need to be cued, prompted, even chaperoned, sometimes, to get back into their roles. They tend to ad lib their way out of sticky situations and flounce off when upstaged. All this when they stick to the script. Imagine what can happen when the virus hijacks the playbook.

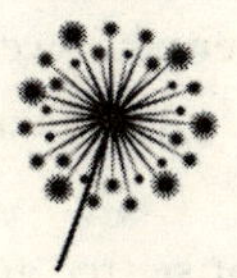

13
The Cleaning Crew

We don't remember what we want to remember,
we remember what we can't forget.

– Lisa Taddeo, *Three Women*, 2019

The airway's first response to an irritant is muco-ciliary clearance.

Mucus is the yucky stuff we sneeze or cough out. It is a gel composed of a glycoprotein called mucin, water and many other molecules. Its production in airway cells is carefully controlled. There are seventeen genes that code for mucin—which tells us just how important it is to the respiratory tract. These genes are tweaked not only by host factors but also by microbes in inhaled air. Imagine that! Viruses and bacteria we inhale can actually manipulate the genes that control an important respiratory defence.

Many molecules in mucus perform anti-microbial activity. The sticky, slithery layer of mucus is secreted to trap and extrude injurious particles from inhaled air. These particles include bacteria, viruses, fungi, air pollutants and toxins.

But that's just the beginning. To extrude these entrapped particles, another form of airway defence comes into play: cilia.

Cilia are minute, hair-like projections on the surfaces of airway cells. They project into the airway, their tips just brushing the secreted mucus. They keep up a rhythmic movement, clear the airway and sweep the mucus upwards at a rate of 5.5 mm/min. Beneath the airway surface layer is a less viscous zone, where the cilia can have free play.

The work of cilia can be affected by a number of factors:

~ Low temperatures slow down ciliary activity—which is why ice cream is a bad idea in the time of COVID-19.

~ Cigarette smoke also makes the cilia's functioning lazier—a good reason to stop smoking now.

~ Dry air makes the cilia inefficient—which is why humidification is sensible.

~ Cilia work best at body temperature. Steam inhalations injure the delicate cilia. It is also a bad idea to drink your beverages scalding hot—if your coffee cup is too hot to be held against your cheek, the coffee is too hot to slosh against your airway.

~ Irritant molecules, like menthol, impede cilia.

~ Rubs, liniments, balms and entire pharmacies of soothing, and very fragrant, decongestants often land up doing the exact opposite. Haven't you gone through the misery of getting a faint trace of pain balm in your eye? Why would you want to singe your respiratory tract with something like that?

So please, in this time of COVID-19, when you reach for that comforting eucalyptus rub or steam kettle—desist! Please let your cilia work.

Defence mechanisms in the airway work brilliantly most of the time. In the presence of irritants, chronic inflammation can set in, changing the scenario. Now, these very efficient defence systems betray the host by going horribly wrong—and actually aid the invading virus.

Our bodies demonstrate a certain degree of 'tolerance', the ability to endure the presence of a pathogen without falling sick. Put another way, tolerance means that we can inhale a heavy viral load and still escape illness. But tolerance is impaired under conditions of constant irritation, which lead to long-standing inflammation within the airway—and bang!—infection.

That's why I think that the strategy against Covid-19 should be weighted on the host, not the virus.

Viruses, even SARS-CoV-2, are everywhere—it is the response of our body that will decide between sickness and health.

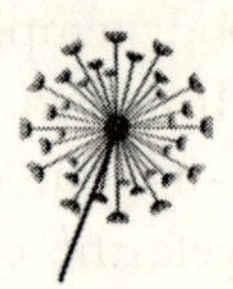

14

The Spike

So! Everything is sentient!

– Pythagorus of Samos, c. 570–c. 495 BCE

How do we recognise this virus? It is displayed everywhere as an angry scarlet ball studded with spikes. This picture feeds into the worst excesses of myth and pseudoscience to reinforce a sense of helplessness in the face of an unseen and pervasive threat.

I see the coronavirus as a crown of thorns. We can choose to respond to its challenge with panic—or we can redeem ourselves with intelligence.

This crown is hollow, but its thorns—spikes of protein with which the virus invades the cell—are real.

The coronavirus spike is not really a spike. It is a club-shaped protrusion with three heads. Structurally, it is a trimeric glycoprotein: it has three binding heads and a membrane-binding stalk. The spike is a fusion protein. It can shuffle its structure to make the virus membrane fuse with the host cell membrane, to facilitate entry.

This distinct structure tells us that the spike employs a double stratagem. It splits into two subunits—S1 and S2 proteins. S1 engages with a receptor site on the host cell. S2 fuses the virus membrane with that of the host.

The spike docks into the host cell by recognising the receptor called ACE2. Once receptor binding is done, the spike protein stabilises itself by shedding the S1 fraction and fusing S2 with the cell membrane. For this to happen, there must be a cleavage of the spike protein. This is accomplished by a protease, a protein-splitting enzyme, present on the host cell.

All coronaviruses use proteases on the host cell for S1-S2 cleavage. Depending on the type of coronavirus and the type of host cell, different proteases may be in play. SARS-CoV-2 uses the host protease furin.

The rest of SARS-CoV-2 is not as spectacular as the spike, but in their quiet way, all parts contribute to infection and, subsequently, to replication.

After binding with the ACE2 receptor, the virus must enter the cell's interior. This is a complex and crowded place. The virus must find a niche to set up its replicating machinery, produce future generations, educate them and send them out into the world.

The fusion of virus and host cell membranes releases viral genome into the cytoplasm. From then, infection of the host involves five steps:

~ choking off the host cell's metabolism
~ copying the virus-RNA
~ replicating the virus genome
~ assembling virions
~ releasing virions from cells

It is a complicated agenda for a pathogen that has no energy currency, no machinery to work with, no workplace.

Not to worry, the host can supply all that!

SARS-CoV-2 shares 98 per cent sequence identity with the spike protein from the bat coronavirus RaTG13, and 76 per cent with SARS-CoV. The SARS-CoV-2 genome has eleven genes. It codes for, at the least, sixteen nonstructural proteins, four structural proteins and a few accessory ones.

The RNA-dependent RNA polymerase (*RdRp*), also known as non-structural protein 12 (nsp 12), is the central component of viral replication. Viral RNA synthesis is achieved by *RdRp*, assisted by other nonstructural proteins (mainly nsp7 and nsp8). *RdRp* also copies viral RNA.

The next step is translation of viral structural proteins, S, E, M and N, all of which are required to produce a structurally complete viral particle.

~ S protein cleaves and binds to the host cell membrane.

~ N protein is needed for virion formation.

~ M protein, working with N and S, completes virion assembly.

~ E protein gives the finishing touch to virions and gets them ready for exit from the host cell.

These structural proteins now enter a way station, which acts as a nursery: the endoplasmic reticulum-Golgi intermediate compartment (ERGIC), where the viral genome gets encapsulated and matures. The next generation is now ready to exit the cell.

This was the story within the infected cell.

But how does a whole chunk of tissue get infected? And why is the virus so destructive?

In some coronaviruses, the spike protein also acts on the cell membrane to make it stick to adjacent cells and form a syncytium. This results in a quick spread of the virus across tissue, because the adherent cells now behave like one giant infected cell. This also hides the virus—and it is able to evade antibodies.

SARS-CoV-2 binds very tightly to the host's ACE2 receptor—it displays an affinity twenty times greater than SARS-CoV had. This is why it is so rapidly destructive in its actions.

The spike protein is a major determinant of virulence as it decides cell entry. It determines tissue destruction because it encourages syncytium formations—instead of only a couple of cells being infected, an entire segment of tissue can be quickly targeted. It also decides 'tissue tropism', that is, which tissues to target and what host to patronise. Both these factors are determined by the availability of ACE2 receptors in the tissue.

Despite the similarity between this new virus that causes Covid-19 and the older SARS virus, there is very weak 'cross-reactivity'. Antibodies produced in response to the SARS-CoV spike protein will not satisfactorily neutralise the SARS-CoV-2 spike protein. In other words, a person who has been infected by the old SARS virus will not necessarily be immune to Covid-19.

There is also another host factor that the spike protein engages with. It is an immunoglobulin, present in the cell membrane, and is called CD147.

CD147 is expressed in inflamed cells, infected cells or cancerous cells. In effect, all sick cells. Healthy cells do not express CD147.

CD147 represents yet another route of entry for the virus. It may turn out to be important as there are drugs which are known to block CD147. Such drugs will bypass normal tissue and reduce chances of an uncontrollable immune response.

The spike protein is vital to the design of vaccines and drugs. Our road to redemption may yet be through this crown of thorns.

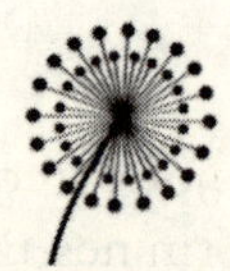

15
Immunity

We're terrible animals. I think that the planet's immune system is trying to get rid of us, and it should.

– Kurt Vonnegut, Jr on 'The Daily Show'

What does it mean to be immune to a disease?

When you're immune to a bug, it can't affect you ever again. It could be bacteria or virus, or perhaps protozoan, helminth or protist.[7] Whatever the bug, if you have lifelong immunity, once bitten, forever shy.

The virus that causes COVID-19 can be inhaled. That takes it straight to the most vulnerable part of the body—the bit of outside we carry inside.

Our lungs are just bags of atmosphere. Even without SARS-CoV-2, the lung is a battlefield. We are oblivious to the skirmishes in there, because we escape unscathed. And that is because of immunity.

A century ago, the immunologist was a magician who provided the elixir of life.

Today, immunologists know that immunity is a double-edged sword.

And never has that been so evident as with COVID-19.

The disease is still unfolding, and many of its puzzles have to do with immunity.

---

7. A protist is any eukaryotic organism (an organism with cells containing a nucleus) that is not an animal, plant or fungus. Protists are part of the biological kingdom called the Protista.

Let me clarify right away that immunity is not something you can 'boost' with an air pump. This folly of new age advertising seems to have arrested all scientific common sense.

In the time of COVID-19, we cannot afford such feel-good nostrums—they are dangerous.

The process that results in immunity is very complex. It has hair-trigger controls.

Immunity comes with the health warning: *Keep Off!*

When a microbe like SARS-CoV-2 is inhaled, the airway's intelligence and defence systems recognise the intruder and react immediately. This is the innate immune response. Non-specific and immediate, it is also very temporary. It leaves no memory of the attack. The next time the same organism is inhaled, the immune response will have to be cranked up again.

Innate immunity is effective but tedious. It works just fine for invertebrates, but ever since we grew ourselves a spine, we have found a more efficient way of defence: this is learnt or adaptive immunity. It is specific to a disease, and if it works, you're cured. It can be switched on at every exposure to that disease, and you won't get the same illness again for a while, perhaps never again. Adaptive immunity is the basis of immunisation with a vaccine.

Innate and adaptive immunity work in tandem, not sequentially, as was thought earlier. They influence each other and use molecules that regulate the process of inflammation.

Immunity is about using inflammation intelligently and effectively.

Two jobs must be accomplished.

First, the infecting organism (pathogen) must be killed or expelled—that's obvious.

The second job of immunity is usually ignored. This is to prevent, or limit, tissue injury. If, in the course of disease, body organs are irreparably injured, they will no longer function, and the patient will die.

Why should this happen?

The weapons of immunity can turn traitor and injure the body itself. These weapons are the chemicals of inflammation.

In COVID-19, where the killer factor is ARDS, the immune process does not, or cannot, use inflammation intelligently.

Most people who are infected with SARS-CoV-2 will recover because the immune process works intelligently.

The weapons of immunity are designed to intercept every step of the virus's progress. And the virus, of course, has developed strategies to counter these.

Every cell in the body is equipped to recognise a pathogen as a harmful intruder; receptors, on the surface and within, recognise molecular patterns that are harmful. Receptors of special importance in viral infections are Toll-like receptors, or TLRs. TLRs are plentiful in mast cells, macrophages and dendritic cells. Mast cells and macrophages initiate the innate immune response, while dendritic cells begin the adaptive response. Once TLRs detect viral protein or RNA, they activate a cascade of molecules to switch on the genes that express chemicals called cytokines.

The name 'cytokine', literally cell-mover, is very apt: cytokines nudge other cells into action. The target could be the very cell that has produced them, and it could lie in surrounding tissue or quite far away.

Cytokines are the chemicals of inflammation. And because their ambit is so wide, their effects in the body are diverse: cytokines can both initiate or stop inflammation.

Their actions are central to the disease process in COVID-19.

The most vital cytokines in viral infections are interferons.

Although interferons are present in health, it takes viral material to prime them up to charge. The moment interferons are released, every cell in the body knows a virus has arrived, a dangerous stranger who has to be locked out. This is a red alert. In response, a slew of genes—300 or thereabouts—are triggered to stop virus replication within the cell. Almost every cell in the body now produces interferons and nudges its neighbour into doing so. There are some cells, special dendritic cells and monocytes, that make interferons their lifework.

Interferons can stimulate cells to express potent antiviral molecules. They can regulate apoptosis. They can stop viral replication. They encourage immune cells to 'present the antigen' to start off the adaptive immune process.

Interferon pathways can be both pro- and anti-inflammatory. For the immune response to be effective, the two arms have to be in balance. The process of inflammation must be halted by anti-inflammatory cytokines before it gets out of hand. The brakes slammed on by anti-inflammatory cytokines terminate the acute response.

But what if this doesn't happen and interferon activity persists?

Tissue destruction is the tragic outcome. Interferons can do this through immunity overdrive.

In COVID-19, this is exactly what happens. The uncontrolled, and uncontrollable, immune reaction pushes the lungs into a state beyond recall:

~ The patient experiences breathlessness and collapse.

~ The doctor diagnoses a failure of oxygenation: ARDS. The outcome may be fatal.

~ The last label for this change in the lung is diffuse alveolar destruction.

This final diagnosis is made by the pathologist who examines the lung tissue under the microscope.

Interferons induce cells to produce molecules called chemokines. These chemicals attract cells. When tissue is exposed to infection or injury, chemokines will attract a contingent of monocytes from the blood. These monocytes immediately express pro-inflammatory factors and aid in the innate immune response. This is a time-limited process, and once it is complete, these cells take a surprising U-turn: they turn into macrophages and clean up dead cells and virus debris. They also secrete a powerful set of anti-inflammatory cytokines to stop the immune response. When this fails to happen, the result is persistent inflammation and aberrant repair processes that lead to tissue damage and fibrosis.

Viruses have evolved strategies to either evade or subvert chemokines. They produce 'fake' chemokine signals to precipitate a drunk and disorderly immune response.

Interferons protect us from viruses whose potential for harm we cannot begin to imagine. We know this from animal experiments: block the production of interferons, and mice will succumb to overwhelming viral infection.

To succeed in infecting us, SARS-CoV-2 must outwit our interferon response.

It is very like a game of chess.

Do viruses have free will?

The thought keeps me awake some nights. But it is consoling too.

The virus doesn't want to kill. It is neither eleemosynary nor minatory—these are human attributes. The virus just wants to replicate and spread.

Immune cells are both immediate and 'learned' responders. Some of them circulate in the blood, others are located in the bone marrow, lymph nodes, liver, kidney and spleen. Yet others are sequestered in various tissues, including the skin.

Neutrophils are immediate responders. They are attracted to the site of infection by pro-inflammatory cytokines, and having arrived, they make short work of the enemy by engulfing and digesting it. Neutrophils are usually killed along with their prey. If scavenger cells (macrophages) are not efficient enough, the detritus of dead neutrophils can severely damage tissue.

Cells infected with viruses are identified and destroyed by lymphocytes called natural killer cells.

Dendritic cells pick up antigens—bits of viral protein—and carry them to nearby lymph nodes, where they present the antigens to lymphocytes and educate them in adaptive immunity.

There are two main groups of adaptive immunity cells:

~ T cells originate in the thymus gland.

~ B cells originate in the bone marrow.

Educated T cells will activate B cells into producing antibody. There are killer T cells too, primed to destroy infected cells. Adaptive immunity is constantly directed, or distracted, by chemokines and cytokines, which either prompt it to act ferociously or caution it to hold back, depending on the virulence of the infection.

Interleukins are a family of cytokines involved in the differentiation and activation of immune cells. Of these, interleukin-6 (IL-6) regulates the innate immune response. In Covid-19 there is a virus-driven increased production of IL-6, which may be responsible for the cytokine storm.

How does immunity alter in Covid-19? Why does the body go into inflammatory overdrive, with massive tissue destruction?

We don't have the answer yet, but the picture is emerging one pixel at a time.

There have been studies of cell types and cytokines that say little more than what is already clinically evident. Some studies implicate one particular cell or one cytokine, only to be displaced soon by another set of observations. All one can say, at this point of time, is that the innate immune response is in free fall. There is prolonged and sustained inflammation, which ends in severe tissue damage.

The lung is not the only target. The cardiovascular system is affected, through disordered inflammation and by direct destruction of heart muscle.

The process of adaptive immunity, which establishes a memory for the antigen, takes time. Memory B and T cells don't take part in the immune response. Once the infection is past, the active B and T cells that battled so hard hang up their swords and undergo apoptosis. Memory cells will stay on in the circulation.

If a second bout of infection from the same virus were to occur, memory cells rapidly clone themselves and exhibit so strong an immune response that the host is often oblivious of ever having been infected.

How long does learnt immune response last?

Sometimes it is lifelong. In the case of quickly mutating viruses, a year.

Against SARS-CoV-1, immunity evidently lasts a year.

Covid-19 presents many challenges, the first of which is the preponderance of ACE2 receptors in the upper airway lining. The nasal mucosa seems to be the principal arena of infection. Mucosal linings—the moist, pink inner walls of the tubes that connect pristine body cavities with the exterior—have their own local immune system. Some infections, like this one, are above their pay grade, and the response is not strong enough to keep the infection from spreading.

Any vaccine, therefore, will have to be directed at this area of extreme vulnerability. We should worry about our lungs, yes, but the nose is nothing to be sneezed at.

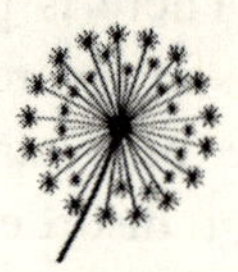

16
The ACE2 Receptor

And like a nascent eye veiled by its lids ...

– Gérard de Nerval, *Selected Writings*, 185
(translated by Richard Sieburth)

We know that the spike docks into the host cell by recognising the receptor called ACE2.

In the general imagination, ACE2 is a Covid-centric, objectionable piece of trash that must be immediately choked off, if we're to stop this pandemic.

'I don't know what the fuss is all about,' a friend told me disapprovingly the other day. 'All they have to do is block off ACE2, and I can't imagine why nobody's done it yet.'

My irate friend is not a virologist. He parted ways with science soon after puberty, and spends his life on the stock market. A self-styled 'information analyst', he sends me Covid-19 analyses every six hours.

'What's ACE2?' I teased. 'What do the letters stand for?'

'I don't know, and I don't care! It is the villain of the piece. Just get rid of it.'

That, really, was the weakness in his analysis.

Angiotensin converting enzyme (ACE) isn't something we can do without.

ACE2, the receptor this virus eagerly hooks up with, what is it?

Every molecule in the body has evolutionary purpose: we have it because we need it. Obviously, ACE2 is not in our cells for the express purpose of attracting coronaviruses.

When you consider that all the tissues in the body simply bristle with ACE2, it is evident that we need a lot of this molecule.

ACE2 is ancient. It has been around for, at least, 518 million years. The oldest form of life known to have ACE2 receptors are annelids—worms. Through our long, slow, blundering climb up the evolutionary ladder, we have clung on to ACE2.

Evolution travels light. It only carries forward genes that adapt us for survival. We wouldn't have held on to something for half a billion years if it weren't vital to our survival as a species.

Ever since we became vertebrates, ACE2 and its antagonistic twin, ACE, have managed our blood pressure and cardiac health. They are the two preeminent stars of a regulatory system that keeps us fit by maintaining a steady blood pressure no matter how diverse our environment. This system, the renin-angiotensin system, controls salt balance, circulating blood volume and, consequently, blood pressure.

Renin is a hormone secreted by the cells of the kidney. Renin activates the hormone angiotensin. Angiotensin is inactive until converted by an enzyme into angiotensin 1 and angiotensin II. We haven't yet worked out what angiotensin I does, but we know a lot about its twin: angiotensin II raises blood pressure.

The enzyme that liberates angiotensin II is ACE. It is antagonised by another molecule, ACE2, which splits angiotensin II into angiotensin 1-7, all molecules that lower blood pressure.

ACE was isolated in 1956, identified then as a 'hypertension-converting enzyme'. It crowds the body. Lungs, intestines, aorta, heart, kidneys—they are all rich in ACE.

The number of ACE and ACE2 receptors in body tissue is much more than could possibly be required to maintain blood pressure. They, obviously, have a wider and more important function.

The gene for ACE2 was isolated in 2000. In humans, it is mapped on the X chromosome. The body tissues with maximum ACE2 receptors are the heart, blood vessels, gut, lungs (particularly in type 2 alveolar cells and macrophages), kidneys, testes and brain. ACE2 crowds the mouth, throat, nasal passages and paranasal sinuses. And it heavily populates adipose tissue, which also contains ACE—that's right, they are just about everywhere.

Recently, researchers analysed the expression of the gene that codes for ACE2 in body tissues. (Increased expression simply means enhanced activity of the molecule the gene codes for.) They found the highest expression in the small intestine, testes, kidneys, heart, thyroid and adipose tissue. The lungs, colon, liver, bladder, adrenal glands were in a middling range, while blood, spleen, bone marrow, brain, blood vessels and muscle had the lowest expression.

Despite the lung having just average amounts of ACE2, it is the killing field in Covid-19.

So what exactly is the role of the ACE2 receptor in this disease?

Alveolar cells have both ACE and ACE2 receptors aplenty. How does this twinned control operate?

SARS-CoV also engages the ACE2 receptor. During the SARS epidemic we learnt some details about how ACE2 acts in the lung. ACE2 is mostly bound to cell membranes. In the healthy body, it rarely circulates in the blood. Raised levels of ACE2 in the blood are only found in disease states.

As we saw earlier, ACE2 converts angiotensin II into angiotensin 1-7. These molecules are strongly anti-inflammatory.

1. ACE2 receptors in the ciliated lining of the airway immobilise an important pro-inflammatory chemical, bradykinin.

2. ACE2 products, angiotensin 1-7, act on receptors on platelets to regulate blood clotting. In the absence of ACE2, microthrombi (small clots) can quickly build up.

3. ACE and ACE2 are present in fat cells. In obesity, when fat deposits increase, ACE2 activity decreases and ACE predominates. This increases the concentration of pro-inflammatory chemicals.

When SARS-CoV-2 spike protein binds with the ACE2 receptor, this molecule is inactivated. It can no longer perform its functions. What is the consequence?

We have answers from experimental studies on isolated lung tissue. The down-regulation of ACE2 injures the lung beyond repair. It produces sustained uncontrollable inflammation. In short—ARDS.

Experimentally, ACE2-knockout mice show an extreme vulnerability to inhaled particulates, tobacco smoke and gastric acid. They quickly succumb to ARDS.

Experimentally isolated SARS-CoV-2 spike protein can directly injure lung tissue by down-regulating ACE2.

This tells us that the therapeutic potential of ACE2 is enormous. Can introducing ACE2 as a drug stop Covid-19 from progressing to the dreaded complication of ARDS?

Researchers have tested a clinical-grade human recombinant soluble ACE2 (hrsACE2) on infected cells in a culture. This hrsACE2 can reduce viral replication in the cultured cells by a significant factor. But it doesn't stop replication entirely.

(This is explained by the possibility of a second mode of viral entry. The choice of this second receptor seems linked with the protease that cleaves the spike protein of this virus.)

Organoids—cells cultured to organise into the organs they were harvested from—can be directly infected by SARS-CoV. Organoid experiments show that SARS-CoV-2 directly infects the walls of the blood vessels, as endothelial or 'inner lining' cells are rich in ACE2 receptors. In these experiments, the organoids treated with hrsACE2 do not get infected.

We will return to the ACE2 receptors when we examine COVID-19's many disastrous effects.

In the lung, ACE2 receptors are principally expressed in type 2 alveolar cells. It is time we took a closer look at them.

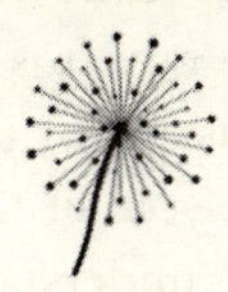

17
Type 2 Alveolar Cells

Si vis pacem, para bellum

– Publius Flavius Vegetius Renatus, *De Re Militari*

Morbidity and Mortality (M&M) are the two most dreaded words in medicine. They cut us down to size, show us exactly how little our vaunted skills accomplish.

M&M meetings are held in the aftermath of clinical conundrums, shockingly unexpected deaths, failed surgeries—or simply, as a weekly routine. The script never varies: a cocky pathologist reads out post-mortem findings, and the resident takes the rap. It is horrible and fascinating, and none of us would miss it for the world. Even if it isn't your case under scrutiny, you sit through it pop-eyed with the greed and the need to understand.

Max Planck, the father of quantum physics, is known for the aphorism 'science advances one funeral at a time'. And indeed, the pathologist holds the key to a world the clinician can only guess at. To learn how little we know, it is only necessary to attend an autopsy—some impressions are indelible.

Ever since Covid-19 broke out, I've found it impossible to dismiss the memory of a post-mortem I witnessed as a young resident. On the slab lay the limp body of a two-year-old who, but an hour ago, had been brought into Casualty, writhing in anguish. The only history the parents could offer was they suspected the child had swallowed kerosene. The mother had drawn a cupful from the keg, left it on the kitchen floor, and gone out to do the washing. When she returned, the toddler was frothing at the mouth, blue in the face—and the cup was empty.

The child died within the hour, and here I was, waiting out the autopsy, quite certain of the diagnosis. The child had choked for certain—death had been too rapid for anything else. When the chest was opened, the reek of kerosene almost knocked me out. I still can't believe what I saw in that chest cavity—total annihilation of the respiratory tract. The collapsed lungs melted at touch into sticky liquefaction.

The child's suffering had been extreme—but even that degree of distress could not have predicted this degree of damage. The rapidity of the child's death had shocked me. Now I wondered what had kept him alive for even that brief hour.

The first reports from Wuhan, with their baffling story of sudden death in mildly symptomatic patients, awakened this memory, and I scanned the internet impatiently in the weeks that followed, for the M&M.

It was a long time coming.

This quote from one of the reports explains why:

> In China, medical autopsies are not commonly performed. In addition, there are special biosafety concerns associated with patients who have died of Covid-19. Therefore, no autopsies could be performed on patients who died of Covid-19 in the early phase of the outbreak. Autopsies were later permitted to be performed under stringent biosafety regulations, but in Wuhan, there is a shortage of autopsy labs meeting these requirements. Faced with these challenges, we sought for alternatives such as the postmortem biopsies used in this study … We recognize that due to limited sampling in needle core

procedures, studies using postmortem biopsies carry certain limitations.

That paragraph reveals, more than anything else, the difficulties faced by these very first responders to a mystifying illness. Despite that modest disclaimer, the post-mortem lung biopsies for COVID-19-related deaths are very telling: they reveal diffuse alveolar destruction, the structural change in the lung in acute respiratory failure.

Diffuse alveolar destruction occurs when the inflammatory process cannot limit itself, and proceeds to squeeze out protein-containing fluid into the alveolar space. A similar structural change is seen in the lungs of people who die of high altitude pulmonary edema. In acute silicosis, where the lung's response to silica can be an overwhelming pneumonia, the structural change is similar.

The most significant change in lung structure in diffuse alveolar destruction relates to the type 2 alveolar cell. Compared to type 1 alveolar cells, which are also found in the bronchioles, type 2 cells are tucked away in the corners and niches of alveolar walls. Type 1 cells are quickly injured—and this is a signal for type 2 cells to proliferate and to substitute, for they act as stem cells.

Type 2 alveolar cells produce surfactant (dipalmitoyl-phosphatidylcholine) to maintain the integrity of the alveolus/capillary unit for effective gas exchange. Without surfactant, the thin walls of the alveolus would collapse on themselves at the end of expiration.

Changes in type 2 alveolar cells may be the vital determinant of lung injury; type 2 cells are impacted in many conditions that end in irreparable lung damage. The most widely studied of such conditions is silicosis, the best kept secret among all environmental diseases. In silicosis, there is an increase in the number and activity of type

2 alveolar cells, leading to the increased production of surfactant.

A number of factors make type 2 alveolar cells central to the complications of Covid-19:

~ They have a very high expression of ACE2 receptors and therefore are viral targets.

~ These cells are rich in molecules that modulate immunity.

~ They have heightened expression of TLRs, which produce a wide spectrum of cytokines.

When the virus engages ACE2 in type 2 alveolar cells, all functions of ACE2 are inhibited. This gives ACE a free rein to exert its pro-inflammatory effects. Surfactant production is altered, in quality and quantity, to increase alveolar collapse. Repair of alveolar cells is no longer possible. Lung injury progresses rapidly. This soon leads to diffuse alveolar destruction.

The M&M on Covid-19 patients is now a daily exercise, and the type 2 alveolar cell will soon take centre-stage.

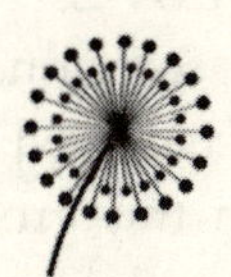

18

The First Cohort

Like diamonds, we are cut with our own dust.

– John Webster, *The Duchess of Malfi*, 1612

41 patients, 1 January–20 January 2020.
Wuhan, Hubei Province, China.

On 31 December 2019, an epidemiological alert was issued. It declared the presence of an infective pneumonia in Wuhan.

On 1 January 2020, the Huanan Seafood Market in Wuhan was sealed off.

By this time, fifty-nine suspected cases, with dry cough and fever, were transferred to the designated Jinyintan Hospital. Of these fifty-nine, forty-one tested positive, on RT-PCR or next generation sequencing, with the virus that is today called the SARS-CoV-2.

This pilot group of forty-one patients represent the spectrum of disease as it emerged:

~ The median age in this group was forty-nine years. There were no children or adolescents.

Fourteen patients were aged between fifty to sixty-four years.

~ In most of them the illness began with fever, cough and body ache.

~ All of them had abnormal findings on chest CT scans, and forty patients had X-ray abnormalities in both lungs—a generalised haziness that resembled a pane of ground glass.

~ All the patients had pneumonia.

Electron microscopy of the airway washings revealed viral particles that bore a typical corona of spikes. The blood picture was consistent with a viral infection.

Thirteen patients developed breathing problems that required intensive care, oxygen and, in four cases, assisted ventilation on a respirator.

Six patients died.

Thirty of these patients were men. Thirteen of them had other illnesses, including diabetes and heart disease.

In those who developed respiratory complications, ARDS set in within two days of hospital admission.

Twenty-seven patients were connected with the Huanan Market. Patients who needed ICU care (thirteen) and those who didn't (fourteen) had the same degree of exposure to the market.

The earliest symptomatic patient had no connection with the Huanan Market at all. He had experienced symptoms since 1 December 2019. His family and contacts had not contracted the illness.

Criteria for discharge from hospital was ten days without fever and an absence of viral particles in nasal and throat swabs.

By 24 January, 835 laboratory-confirmed infections were reported in China, with twenty-five dead.

By this time, person-to-person infection had been established.

COVID-19 had these distinct features:

a. Upper airway symptoms were negligible: there were very few runny noses and productive coughs.
b. SARS and MERS patients frequently had abdominal complaints of pain and diarrhoea. That was not seen in this cohort.

c. The terminal complication of ARDS was accompanied by an abnormal cytokine profile—suggestive of the 'cytokine storm' that is encountered in SARS, MERS and a number of other septic states.

This was the picture at the onset of the epidemic.

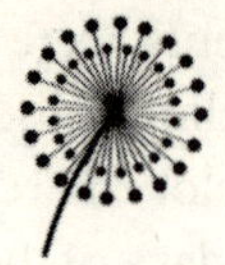

19
Inflammation

He who learns must suffer. And even in our sleep pain that cannot forget falls drop by drop upon the heart, and in our own despair, against our will, comes wisdom to us by the awful grace of God.

– Aeschylus, *Agamemnon*, first performed 458 BCE

Inflamed is an emberous word. Red hot, it threatens injury. *Keep Off!* it warns.

It also hints at a certain moral weakness. By being *inflamed* one has, somehow, reneged on social obligations. No longer trustworthy, inflamed is midway between embarrassment and menace.

Its origin is easily guessed: *in flamma.* I like to read that as 'inner fire'. But is it a fire that energises, or one that destroys?

Hippocrates and his gang on Kos, circa 350 BCE, noticed inflammation as a red, swollen and painful body part. Touched, it felt warm even though the patient was not running a fever. Several hundred years later, a Roman physician, Celsus, wrote down those impressions in four immortal words that every medical student today inherits: *Rubor, Calor, Dolor, Edema.*

Which is merely Latin for what is common knowledge in any language: when a body part is inflamed, it is red, hot, painful and swollen.

'Inflamed' runs the gamut of a love story: anger, pleasure, obsession, betrayal, danger. Tragedy. *Romeo and Juliet*, entire.

The human experience of inflammation begins way ahead of redness, heat, swelling and pain. We hardly ever notice our bodies through the busy day, but there is a state when the body intrudes on our consciousness. When it hangs about and nags for attention. When a white noise burgeons in volume and distracts until it dislocates.

That is the experience of inflammation before you get red hot and swollen and feel actual pain.

Inflammation is a state of awareness.

I have relied on this definition ever since the first reports of COVID-19 came in, before it was even called COVID-19. From the very first patients, the unnamed three who coughed out the virus, COVID-19 revealed the spectrum of inflammation, this state of awareness.

Dry nagging cough.

Exhaustion.

Before that, mild fever and the sense that something wasn't quite right.

Then came the illness.

Doctor and patient have diametrically opposite views about illness.

The patient experiences illness as unnatural, as body failure, because the body's natural state is health. The doctor, on the other hand, observes illness, detached from the experience of it. Illness is observed as signs. The doctor sees illness as body response.

And most of these responses are part of the spectrum of inflammation. Cough is a mechanical response to irritation. When it persists, think of a state of constant irritation, enough to get you spitting mad. And you *do* spit. Because the 'you' that's inflamed is a tissue that produces secretions—the respiratory tract. Fever is a chemical response to irritants. The chemicals are the molecules of inflammation, dozens of them.

Again, the patient perceives fever as dangerous, while the doctor perceives fever as protective. Within limits, fever—the 'heat' of inflammation—signals cellular fight back. It is inflammation's clarion call for reinforcements.

Our three patients at Wuhan Jinyintan Hospital experienced shortness of breath—the key symptom of COVID-19. Thereafter, their paths diverged:

Guan-Yin got worse before she recovered.

Jiān succumbed.

Bohai recovered without much suffering.

To understand that, we will have to consider the *site* of inflammation: the airway.

Consider again the basic design of the airway: a tube that ends in a teabag swishing around in blood.

The site of inflammation in COVID-19 is the lower airway—and the walls of that teabag. Time now we called that teabag by its proper name: alveolus.

Hundreds of alveoli, considered together, make up a lung, and we have two of them. That is a lot of space for air. When we are well, breathing is so easy we never notice it. But it takes effort, just the same.

When Guan-Yin, Jiān and Bohai felt a shortness in their breathing, it was because their muscles had to work harder to fill and empty their lungs.

Why would that happen?

The instinctive answer is the right one (usually)—the lungs have become heavier, and therefore difficult to move. From being filmy bags, full of air, they have become thick-walled sacs, congested with the liquid products of inflammation.

Bohai's lungs cleared quickly, and the inflammatory fluids drained away. This is inflammation at its optimum—protective and efficient.

In Guan-Yin, inflammation was stretched to the limit. She continued to suffer because the walls of her lungs grew stiff due to the swelling and, therefore, inelastic. Her muscles laboured on nonetheless, biding time until the fluid drained away. Throughout her illness, her lungs continued to work because gas exchange had still been possible across those thick inflamed walls.

But Jiān's lungs were hit much harder, and inflammation went into overdrive. The thickened walls of his beleaguered lungs became leaky, the alveolar space that should have contained only air became a dirty puddle of inflammatory liquids and dead cells. Gas exchange dropped to levels that verged on the dangerous. Breathing became nearly impossible—his lungs were now solid. The effort of filling and emptying was beyond Jiān's tiring muscles. He could no longer breathe on his own, so he was put on assisted ventilation. The machine delivered oxygen under positive pressure to each thick puddle in his lung. But it failed to oxygenate his blood.

Jiān died in hospital, in intensive care, while on a ventilator. But, for all intents and purposes, he drowned in a swamp of injurious chemicals of an uncontrolled and uncontrollable inflammation.

Hippocrates would have recognised this spectrum of suffering.

So would Sushruta, Charaka and Ibn Sina.

So would John Hunter and William Osler.

So does your family doctor.

None of them would have thought to call it Covid-19. None of them may have seen SARS-CoV-2 face-to-face, but all of them would have recognised the process, the damage.

They would have understood that the body's protective responses had slipped the leash. This could no longer be called just 'inflammation'.

Inflammation in the airway is what makes Covid-19 such a frightening disease. It is the disordered response of our own bodies.

What is this response like when it is orderly?

What do redness, heat, pain and swelling actually achieve?

Surely, by now, we must know more than Hippocrates and that entire crowd of ancients?

That is debatable, but one thing is true: we do have many more facts. So, let us try fitting them into these cardinal signs.

Redness, swelling, pain and heat are the result of a complex array of chemicals in the inflammatory process. These chemicals are released in a cascade by a variety of cells, producing the familiar local effects. But inflammation extends beyond the point of injury or infection; it may involve other body systems as well when help is recruited to complete the innate immune response.

An efficient response needs:

~ A way to detect injury or infection.

~ A way to get rid of the intrusion.

~ A way to limit tissue injury or infection from spreading.

~ A way to initiate healing and repair.

With such a complicated agenda, it is only expected that the rest of the body must participate. So, in addition to local factors, messengers are needed to recruit aid. These messengers are chemical and cellular. Because the chemicals and cells of inflammation can be transported by the bloodstream, their effects are perceived in the body's outposts, far removed from the site of action. Inflammation becomes then a systemic response, involving several body functions.

When we considered immunity, we met TLRs, the canny receptors that recognise viral intruders as non-self. TLRs, a family of ten molecules, are vital to the inflammatory response. They start off the process of inflammation by the release of pro-inflammatory cytokines. These cytokines, like IL-1β, IL-6, TNF-α, are released from immune cells: monocytes, lymphocytes, macrophages.

Inflammatory cytokines are cell recruiters—they direct white blood cells to the site of infection or injury. They're kept in check by the anti-inflammatory cytokines. This interaction is vital to maintaining the delicate balance of inflammation. When it gets out of hand, the result is a cytokine storm, unbridled inflammation that can cause massive tissue destruction and a fatal outcome. This is, very likely, the fatal complication in Covid-19.

In addition to these chemical cascades and signalling molecules, oxidative stress can induce the production of reactive oxygen species and reactive nitrogen species. These can increase the expression of genes that code for inflammatory cytokines and chemokines.

So how does this complex orchestra play out the symphony of inflammation?

Let's relate them to the experience of our three core patients of Covid-19.

Fever

Fever is the result of an interplay between immune factors and the established temperature-control system. After TLRs recognise infection, prostaglandin E2 (PGE2) is secreted. This molecule crosses the blood-brain barrier and induces a rise in body temperature.

Neutrophils are then recruited to the site of injury. When it is the lung, as in Covid-19, this is not good news, as the intense reactive oxygen species induced in these cells threaten the integrity of the alveolar wall. To balance this out, fever activates dendritic cells, which hurry up the adaptive immune response.

Cough

Cough is the response to the irritation caused by an inflamed airway. The 'redness' element of inflammation is the result of increased blood flow to the site of infection.

The walls of small arteries dilate due to the action of chemicals (bradykinin, histamine, prostaglandins) released from mast cells, macrophages and endothelial cells. Nitrous oxide, released from endothelial cells further relaxes the vessel wall. These effectually deliver a rush of blood, teeming with immune cells primed to destroy the pathogen.

These inflammatory chemicals are strong airway irritants and induce a persistent cough.

Difficulty in breathing

The work involved in breathing increases as the lung wall grows thick with swelling (edema). This is the result of local effects of the innate immune response.

Inflammatory chemicals set up a boggy swelling in the alveolar wall. Very soon, the cells begin to leak, and the fluid between cells drains into the alveolar space. What should be full of air is now full of sticky proteinaceous fluid.

For the patient to recover, the process of inflammation must subside. Naturally one expects the lung to have a tight system of inflammatory control.

Why doesn't it?

If inflammation is such an evolutionary benefit, how does it go so terribly wrong in COVID-19?

Innate immunity has a very long memory. Invertebrates, even the humblest of them, seem to have honed it to a fine art. They have all the smarts: the cells and the cascades of chemical reactions that produce defence molecules; cytokines; and also all those effector molecules that strike us as such a sophistication when they play out in our own human script. Reactive oxygen and nitrogen species, antimicrobial peptides, lectins, complement-related proteins—worms have them all. Starfish have the most impressive defence against a wide range of pathogens, and all this without adaptive immunity.

Adaptive immunity first appears in vertebrates. As of 2020, the line between these two systems of immunity has blurred considerably. We know that they feed into each other. We also know that they come under genetic control, and individual defects in these genes can determine our susceptibility to infection. Tomorrow's medicine may work on these intelligences and diagnose not disease itself but our ability or inability to recover from it—that would be thrilling. But we still have to make it to that tomorrow. Faced with COVID-19 and the escalating number of the dying and the dead, will we?

In viral infections, the most energetic molecules are TLRs. In the airway, TLRs are present on many immune cells:

alveolar and interstitial macrophages, dendritic cells, airway epithelial cells, innate lymphocytes and neutrophils. Besides these surface receptors, there are receptors inside the cell too. These may have a special role to play in SARS-CoV-2 infection.

Recognition of an RNA virus by TLRs is immediate. This recognition sparks off a cascade of reactions that activate type I/III interferons and a pro-inflammatory gene programme.

Type I interferons activate more than a thousand genes in immune cells and a core group of genes across all cell types. This broad activation is synchronised to stop viral replication and viral spread from cell-to-cell across the tissue. The virus is stopped at every point of its intracellular sojourn, preventing its replication and assembly.

For this to be as precise and infallible as it usually is, the process must be tightly controlled—and so it is. A spectrum of local reactions make certain the innate immune response does not go over the top and result in cellular damage.

Of the interferons, type III interferons, or lambda interferons, are the first line of defence in a viral blockade. They are present on all cells that line the airway. If they prove ineffective, type I interferons are whistled up. This observation was made in the aftermath of the SARS epidemic of 2002–03 and could be of great importance now, with Covid-19. While type III interferons do not tip the inflammatory response into overdrive, type I interferons can.

The complications of Covid-19 are brought about by an unfettered and destructive inflammatory response, which leads up to ARDS.

Immune cells are a scary bunch. They accomplish miracles, but they can turn treacherous without notice.

The first cell to respond to infection is the neutrophil.

Neutrophils appear stippled when you look at them under a microscope. These dots are toxic granules—fours kinds, and each lethal to anything recognised as a pathogen. Despite this finesse, the neutrophil's first card is brute force: it simply engulfs the pathogen by opening wide its ameboid arms. And now comes the baffling bit. This is a suicide mission that the neutrophil goes about with ruthless efficiency. It hides the engulfed pathogen and packs it up swiftly. Shrink-wrapped, the captured prey will not leak out. The neutrophil then enters apoptosis. During apoptosis, those toxic granules stay zip-locked, and the nucleus curls up into another neat packet. The entire neutrophil is now ready to be carted away by a macrophage. If apoptosis is delayed or ineffective, the neutrophil, in its dying throes, will damage surrounding tissue.

Macrophages should be swarming around by this point—but what if they aren't? If the apoptosed neutrophil is left where it is, that neat packaging soon gives way, and those toxic granules leak out and do damage.

This isn't all bad. The local reaction it induces tends to wall off the site of infection. Walls rise as capillaries collapse and lymphatics are blocked. This swelling limits the infection.

Meanwhile, if the pathogen is too big or difficult to be swallowed whole, the neutrophil sets out another trap—a web of fine fibrils that enmeshes the intruder. At the end of this process, too, the neutrophil dies.

It is obvious that the efficiency of immunity's neutrophil response depends not just on the actions of this particular cell but, equally, on the other cells that must arrive in time to clear the field. Neutrophils also 'present' the trapped infecting organism as an 'antigen' to prompt the adaptive immune response.

It appears now that neutrophils could be the key to the complications in Covid-19.

With such a fine-tuned and complex agenda, is it surprising that slip-ups can occur? And, everything that can go wrong does so in Covid-19.

The clearing of neutrophil apoptosis in the lung may be the factor that decides between a mild viral illness and a severe one.

The lung is a very specialised organ: it exhibits a 'global' response to prolonged inflammation from any cause. Covid-19 is lethal because of this response.

But this response is also seen in chronic lung inflammation from many, many conditions—the co-morbidities you have been hearing about—and recognising this might help in identifying the most vulnerable patients.

Why should inflammation be prolonged at all? What signals fail the lung?

If the neutrophil is vital to inflammation in the lung, another kind of cell is integral to maintaining the lung in a steady state of health. This is the alveolar macrophage.

Think of the colourless, mostly odourless, non-irritant stuff we consider clean air—AQI below 50, low in particulates and smoke. It is, besides, unarguably bright; the sky a Hockney blue. Air doesn't get clearer than that blue.

It is still filthy.

A zillion things we couldn't imagine, leave alone see or smell, crowd the atmosphere. A list of toxins alone would run into libraries. And then there are allergens and ultra-fine particles and, yes, microbes, bacteria, fungi, protists.

And viruses.

We inhale and exhale viruses all the time. Yet our lungs stay blissfully healthy.

And all because of the action of alveolar macrophages.

Alveolar macrophages are on 'lung protection' duty from their very first week of life. They're pretty overworked. They recognise pathogens, encourage phagocytosis and clean up after. They remove oxidised lipids from the polluted air we inhale, by expressing the macrophage receptor with collagenous structure (MARCO) gene. They also present antigens to T cells for adaptive immunity. Because of their opposing actions of a) killing pathogens and b) maintaining tissue integrity and promoting repair, alveolar macrophages are considered as two distinctive groups.

By clearing away apoptotic neutrophils, macrophages start off the release of anti-inflammatory factors, to halt the process of inflammation. But this immunosuppressive action of the macrophage can boomerang by allowing pathogens to persist, sequestered from immune surveillance, thus setting the stage for chronic inflammation.

At the beginning of February 2020, we believed that Covid-19 targeted the elderly. Most of the deaths were in people over sixty-five. Children were unaffected by the disease. It almost felt as if a force of nature had decided to purge our ageing population.

By early March, we had hastily revised those impressions. Many young people had succumbed. Even in the first wave of infection, children had not escaped.

Still, the elderly are definitely more vulnerable to the complications of Covid-19, as they are to most respiratory infections. A large part of the disease burden in the 'over sixty-five' age group is respiratory illnesses. This is also the group with a heavy burden of other illnesses: diabetes, cardiovascular disease, arthritis, autoimmune diseases, cancers.

We take it for granted that age is a factor to be considered when examining the outcome of any illness. It is only natural that the ageing body should cave in quicker. We will be condemned for saying it, but it seems the decent thing to do. In ancient cultures, it was a social obligation on the elderly to die. In our day, this is echoed in the cruelty, neglect and social isolation that most elderly people have come to accept as their lot.

All social beliefs, especially morally repugnant ones, are based on truths that relate to the body. So let us overlook attitudes and get to the real thing.

The worst complication of COVID-19 is respiratory failure, a tragic picture of inflammation gone rogue.

Is there any science behind the impression that the elderly are especially vulnerable to COVID-19?

The future is now ... That phrase usually applies to the very elderly. Today, it cuts across all barriers of age.

I think the shifting view of the relationship between age and vulnerability to COVID-19 complications is of great relevance. There is no doubt that the aged are especially vulnerable. That same vulnerability extends to the young too.

Let's start by looking at why older people seem targeted by this virus.

How long are we expected to live anyway?

That is an evolutionary question; it isn't rhetoric.

Is increased vulnerability to disease really a sign that time is running out? Or is it the messed-up part of a new equipment kit? Evolution sneaks upon us unnoticed, and the body adapts in many ways, and immunity is one of them.

Immunity changes as we age. To put it briefly, adaptive immunity becomes sluggish, and our innate immunity is constantly on the defensive. This produces a grumbling state of inflammation, unkindly termed 'inflammaging'.

The thymus gland, the mysterious but powerful generator of the T cells needed in adaptive immunity, ages gracefully in a process called involution and dwindles to a shadow of its former self. That isn't a purely human thing. It seems to happen in all vertebrates, so evolution has conserved this change for—literally—ages.

T cells, 'naïve T cells' have to be ready, when presented with an antigen. to enter the combat mode of adaptive immunity, and the T cells that now trickle out of the ageing thymus are not up to scratch.

We have begun to realise that external factors, not just chronological ageing, contribute to thymic involution.

The lack of competent T cells, as a result of thymic involution, makes adaptive immunity uncertain in the elderly, and this makes them prone to excesses of innate immunity gone rogue. But is this the complete picture?

More elderly people die of noncommunicable illnesses than of infections. Yet their bodies do display an immune response when vaccinated against disease.

How do we explain this paradox?

In evolutionary terms, thymic involution may just be a mechanism to cut down on energy costs. Why keep an organ functioning when it is no longer strictly necessary? Then again, why does it stop being necessary? What assumes its function?

The answer lies in the over-ready innate immune system in the elderly, which makes the thymus redundant. Innate immunity is quick to react, and it reacts strongly. It can easily tip into overdrive and cause fatal complications, as in COVID-19.

The reason for this rapid and enthusiastic response is that the ageing body is already in the pro-inflammatory state of inflammaging—a state defined by co-existing conditions like diabetes, metabolic syndrome, cardiovascular disease, arthritis.

Is the rest of our population—the middle-aged, the ferociously young and even children—in some manner, also inflammaged?

Is there a common denominator?

There is.

It is called the microbiome. Specifically, the gut microbiome.

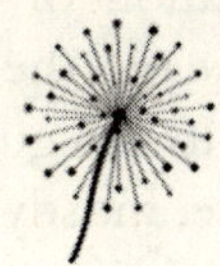

20

The Microbiome

What we excrete comes back to consume us.

– Don DeLillo, *Underworld*, 1997

It is time we noticed the role the microbiome might be playing in Covid-19.

The microbiome, more correctly the human microbiome, is a catch-all term for the trillions of microbes that inhabit our bodies. These bacteria are determinants of how the body functions in health and in disease. Every part of the body has its own population of microbes, including the sacrosanct brain. When we use the term in connection with illness, it generally refers to the gut microbiome—the flora that colonises the intestine, mostly the colon.

It is the gut microbiome that calls all the shots.

Sounds incredible?

Think of the gut microbiome as a supermarket that stocks the stuff needed to maintain cell function at an optimum. Here are a few things that happen there to keep the rest of the body's machinery on its toes:

It converts complex plant carbohydrates in the diet into short chain fatty acids (SCFAs). SCFAs are not only essential sources of energy for the intestinal lining but also have a strong anti-inflammatory effect.

It regulates the fat metabolism. When this is dysregulated, the result is obesity.

It synthesises vitamins.

The immune process is equipped at different stages by a series of small molecules produced here. With special reference to inflammation, immune cells are controlled by signals from the microbiome. As discussed earlier, macrophages can be tuned as pro-inflammatory or anti-inflammatory. The healthy microbiome can activate the 'Warburg Effect'[8] in macrophages. This accumulates intermediate molecules (succinate, fumarate, malate) that modulate immunity.

Alterations in the microbiome—the technical term is dysbiosis—result in disease. More precisely, dysbiosis is an imbalance between 'good' and 'bad' bacteria. This leads to a build-up of microbial products and metabolites that work as irritants and activate the resident macrophages into an inflammatory profile. The result—you guessed it—is chronic inflammation.

The implications of this chronic inflammation are nothing short of staggering, so I'll just take a deep breath and say it—the whole range of metabolic and degenerative diseases: obesity, metabolic syndrome, diabetes, arthritis, autoimmune diseases, cardiovascular disease, Parkinson's, Alzheimer's, multiple sclerosis, inflammatory bowel diseases, cancers ... all diseases with an underlay of chronic inflammation.

As a risk factor, obesity is a pro-inflammatory state. It increases inflammatory mediators IL-6 and TNF-α. Obesity reduces levels of adiponectin, which is anti-inflammatory. It alters local immune cells and maintains a steady state of inflammation across all tissues.

---

8. The German doctor and physiologist Otto Heinrich Warburg was nominated for the Nobel Prize forty-seven times in his career. He won it in 1931 for his discovery of the nature and mode of action of the respiratory enzyme. Born to Protestant parents, but because of his father's Jewish ancestry, he was considered Halbjude, half-Jew, Mischling, mixed-blood (Aryan and Jew) and, finally, Gleichstellung, equal with Aryan Germans as his fame grew.

One third of the global population is obese.

Dysbiosis causes, and sustains, obesity.

What is the link between Covid-19 and the microbiome?

A large number of people who have suffered the fatal complication of respiratory failure in Covid-19 had 'co-morbidities', which means they were already suffering from other diseases when they caught this infection. The chart below shows the number of people of different age groups who had underlying illnesses when they died of Covid-19 in New York in mid-April. The reports about critically ill and fatal cases from other parts of the world are no different: people with illnesses characterised by chronic inflammation are at a definite risk for developing complications from Covid-19.

Inflammaging is no longer ageist. Life on the planet is a constant state of alarm.

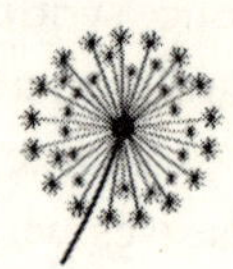

Age	*Number of deaths*	*Share of deaths*	*With underlying conditions*	*Without underlying conditions*	*Unknown if with underlying conditions*	*Share of deaths of unknown and without conditions*
0–17 years old	3	**0.04 per cent**	3	0	0	0 per cent
18–44 years old	309	**4.5 per cent**	244	25	40	1.0 per cent
45–64 years old	1,581	**23.1 per cent**	1,343	59	179	3.5 per cent
65–74 years old	1,683	**24.6 per cent**	1,272	26	385	6.0 per cent
75+ years old	3,263	**47.7 per cent**	2,289	27	947	14.2 per cent
TOTAL	**6,839**	100 per cent	5,151	137	1,551	24.68 per cent

Source: *New York City Health, 14 April 2020*

21
A Timeline

Mene Mene Tekel Upharsin

– *The Book of Daniel*, Chapter 5,
the Septuagint version, c. 100 BCE

We humans code a whole lot of genes for inflammation, many more than our cousin the chimpanzee. More, too, than our putative ancestors, the Denisovans and Neanderthals.

Why do we need so many?

Why inflammation?

We think of the genome as inheritance—which it certainly is—but inheritance of *what?*

The evolving mythology around population genetics feeds into our greed for privilege and control, couched in the familiar guise of race, caste, creed, culture. Or, if you prefer the big word, *civilisation.*

It is time, again, to bring that little pin to this notion. Our genome is nothing so inflated. It is merely a record of circumstance; a memory of daily necessities as mundane—and as anxious—as a shopping list in this time of Covid-19. And, like all shopping lists, it keeps changing.

Yet, throughout time, the two great threats to human existence haven't really changed, have they? They are—and remain—disease and starvation.

To have a life, we must somehow avoid these threats.

In 2019, two-thirds of humanity could not, did not.

Now, in 2020, it appears as if the privileged one-third won't either.

Disease and starvation threaten all of us, for COVID-19 will leave behind poverty on an epic scale. The choice will be ours. We can retreat into the brutish passivity of social isolation and continue to indulge in mindless cruelties that have become the norm: domestic violence, religious separatism, racism, hate. Or, we can respond as a species, with the energy and enlightenment that have made us the most intelligent beings on the planet. Birth is an accident, but thanks to a generous insurance from the genome, we can live a willed existence.

Our cellular pantry is well-stocked against threats of both disease and starvation. To combat disease, the genome encodes inflammation. To combat starvation, it encodes fat. Although these genes are, at the least, 50,000 years old, their effects influence our response to COVID-19.

But the genome isn't a full-grown body part we're stuck with. It is shaped and tutored by circumstance. I like to think of it as an intelligent response to circumstance.

We are, long before we are born, a part of our changing environment. The genome, predictably, will respond to change by up-regulating those genes that code for advantage and down-regulating those that might spell disaster. These responses are dictated by environmental factors that threaten existence, and encompass much more than a handful of germs. These are factors in our external milieus, everything we've been exposed to. This has earned itself a predictable name—the exposome, the nature of nurture. This term was defined by Christopher Wild, in 2005, as 'the totality of human exposures throughout life'.

The body's responses are a record of the changing exposome it faces through its career: from its beginnings as pre-fertilisation parental gametes to the moment of death. Obviously, the exposome has changed through the ages.

Our lungs record that change; the fatal ARDS of COVID-19 has been a long while in the making.

About 5 million years ago, when were still pre-*Homo*, a dry spell caused the lush tropical forests of Africa to thin out into a savannah. This practically forced bipedalism on us. As fruit trees disappeared, we had to walk long distances to find food. Our lungs grew larger to equip us for so much aerobic exercise.

The forest was replaced by savannah. Sharing the table with us now were ungulates, rodents and other odorous riff-raff. Besides pollen from the savannah, we breathed in spores and microbes from animal faeces. The wind blew in fine silica dust from the denuded savannah. All these were 'foreign' particles, allergens.

Fast forward to 10,000 BCE, when villages were established and animals domesticated. By this time, we early humans—always big on art—had begun cutting and polishing stones into jewellery. That called for quarrying—and tool-making. We were being masons when we weren't lapidarists. We were potters when we weren't being sculptors. And the rest of us were farmers and weavers. The estimated global population then was less than 10 million.

Soon after, cities were formed. Work was organised into guilds. Societies were structured. What were we breathing then? This was still a pre-industrial age, one that was very strongly agricultural. Domestication of animals was now rife. This introduced our lungs to a whole new world of animal pathogens. In addition, allergens from plant pollens diversified. Our numbers increased and population density guaranteed a quick transfer of pathogens and particulate matter that could be inhaled, setting the stage for the first recorded epidemics.

Indoor coal and wood fires, particularly in cold climates, increased particulate matter. Stones were broken, ores were mined, metals smelted, jewellery carved and polished. Silica and smoke were everywhere. The human presence was defined by them.

Yes, the airway was saved from all these irritants as long as innate immunity acted responsibly. Illnesses were pathogen-caused. We have, from this time on, a dedicated record of plagues across all cultures. How does all this matter to us now in the time of Covid-19?

The air we breathe today is thick with particulate matter—that is the price we pay for industrialisation and our fossil fuel addiction. In addition to microbes from animals and each other, our kitchen smoke is rich in polycyclic aromatic hydrocarbons and advanced glycation end products.

We breathe in these irritants and still thrive, because by now we have a suite of genes that detoxify the chemicals in domestic smoke. We even have a gene that deals with the chemicals in roasted meat.

By now, we've long perfected the mechanism of innate immunity. We have also acquired a vast group of virus-interacting proteins—which means we have been engaging with viruses for a very long time. In the lungs, working overtime, is a special cell whose job is to present antigen.

We acquired this survival kit pre-Holocene, 12,000 years ago.

With the increase in air pollutants, our sustenance became a high sugar, high fat diet. We now grew fat we no longer needed as an inbuilt larder.

We have been primed with chronic inflammation since the time the industrial age began. Its effects were soon disastrous. The 'Age of Exploration', with its genocide of the Americas and the enslavement of Africa, resulted in another admixture of pathogens. Killer diseases emerged year after year in this period of conquest and colonisation.

These past two hundred years, our chronic inflammation has been driven by pollution in the exposome and fat depots in the body.

What are the major drivers of disease in our own lifetime?

We only have to look at the external milieu of capitalism and the internal milieu of consumerism to understand.

With every breath, these conspire to make us sitting targets for every new infection.

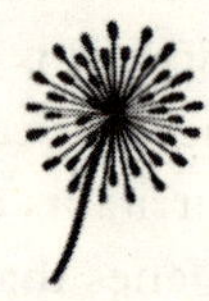

22
Of Mice and Men

And cold sweat holds me and shaking
grips me all, greener than grass
I am and dead—or almost
I seem to me.

– Sappho, *Fragment 31*
(translated by Anne Carson, 2002)

Is SARS-CoV-2 misandrist?

There is a definite preponderance of men in cases with complications.

Are men more prone to ARDS?

Or susceptible to the virus itself?

Or is this just another illusion in the shifting pattern of this disease?

Men and women are equally susceptible to the disease. But at any age, men seem to suffer a more serious illness. (This may still be illusory, as the variables are so many.)

The SARS-CoV-2 spike engages with the ACE2 receptor, which is coded by a gene on the X chromosome. One possibility is that women, blessed with XX, have ACE2 in failsafe quantities even in the presence of a virus that binds tight to the molecule. Men, with XY chromosomes, are not so lucky.

Another possibility is that women have a more protective renin-angiotensin system.

Perhaps this bit of lab wisdom holds a clue. In an experiment, mice, of both genders, were maintained on high-fat meals.

The males grew obese and hypertensive. The females gained weight, but their blood pressure stayed normal.

Obesity, we know, shifts the ACE/ACE2 balance in favour of ACE, thus setting off high blood pressure.

When the obese male mice were given losartan, an ACE inhibitor, they regained normal blood pressure. Since the issue was easily corrected by an ACE-blocker, it indicated that obesity had indeed caused an uptick in ACE, leading to hypertension.

As this didn't happen in female mice, it began to look as if ACE2 was still in charge, despite obesity.

It appears that this difference in response is due to the protective effect of oestrogen, because mice without ovaries behave quite differently. Their responses are … male.

Can this be extrapolated to the human situation? Are women protected by their hormones against the worst excesses of COVID-19?

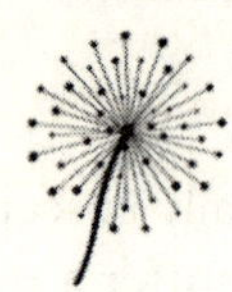

23

I Am Legion

And he asked him, What is thy name? And he answered, saying,
My name is Legion: for we are many.

– Mark 5:9, King James Bible

How do I love thee? Let me count the ways.
I love thee to the depth and the breadth and the height
My soul can reach…

Tuberculosis shadowed Elizabeth Barrett Browning's life. Did she unconsciously transcribe the voice of *Mycobacterium tuberculosis* in that lovely sonnet?

The travails of tuberculosis require more than fourteen lines. The disease demands the magnificent overarching thunder of Milton's *Paradise Lost*, for there is no depth or height or breadth of the human body that it does not seduce.

Tuberculosis converts the depth of bone into a living death, the lingering decay of osteomyelitis. Splinters of bone make a slow voyage to the surface, flotsam in the relentless drip of pus. The breadth of skin is a scribble-board for mycobacteria. Warts, scabby growths, lumps, bumps, white and red dots—tuberculosis does them all, each with a fancy name.

The signature of tuberculosis resembles a crumble of cheese, Pecorino Romano for choice.

Nineteenth-century medicine was big on gastronomy. By 1868, quite ignoring the fact that tubercular crumbles were the detritus of dead tissue packed close, British physicians were calling the phenomenon 'caseation', after the Latin word for cheese. It is an unbeatable simile: caseating lymph nodes slice like brie. And tuberculosis caseates everywhere. The lungs are its most favoured canvas.

Forty years ago, general hospitals in India were libraries of pulmonary tuberculosis—I browsed through one when it was well past its prime. We had drugs by then, and the beds were mostly taken up by dead-end disease. We thought ourselves past that nightmare. Then, thirty years later, tuberculosis did a U-turn and slammed us anew. Multi-drug resistant TB is here to stay: in our guts and genitals, in our livers and kidneys, and cruellest of all, in our brains. It spares none. At each station in life, it lays waste the organs most vital to that age. It is back to its ancient avatar: consumption, kshaya rog, the wasting disease.

Tuberculosis was the most diverse disease we knew. And then came COVID-19.

Six months into the pandemic, COVID-19 was a very far cry from what the index patients in Wuhan experienced. To build the profile of the disease, every case is relevant.

Transparency is paramount. Until we learn what the disease looks like in our neck of the woods, how will we recognise it? The crepuscular public advisory of symptoms—cough, fever, sore throat—is pathetically incomplete.

Doctors everywhere await details from the frontlines to deliver the best care to their own patients. The features described in this chapter are from close encounters over the past months. We may yet be ambushed by completely different presentations in the months ahead.

1. When Kidneys Fail

In a study of 701 COVID-19 patients hospitalised in a critical care facility in Wuhan, 40 per cent were found to have severe kidney disease. Some of them, older men, had signs of kidney affliction on admission, but most developed it in hospital. Many of them died.

Were their kidneys targeted by the virus?

Kidney tissue is rich in ACE2. Perhaps viral entry caused severe kidney damage. Or the damage could have been through those pathways of unbridled inflammation that caused ARDS in these patients.

Is kidney failure part of the general state of severe illness, or can we expect COVID-19 to cause specific kidney damage and therefore manifest as kidney disease or acute kidney failure?

Kidney tissue from patients who died of COVID-19 has revealed extensive damage to the renal architecture.

Viral particles were seen in segments of tissue which are normally rich in ACE2. This is proof of direct tissue destruction by the virus and sufficient to explain kidney failure even in the absence of contributory factors like diabetes and hypertension.

So, yes, SARS-CoV-2 does directly damage kidney tissue. This is in addition to the beating these organs take as part of the general state of shock, inflammation and cytokine storm in severe COVID-19.

2. The First Whiff

When I have a cold, I begin the day with irritation. The most precious part of my day—the first cup of coffee—is utter ruin. No matter how carefully brewed, how airy its froth, how creamy the mouthfeel, coffee tastes flat when I have a cold. Not stronger brew, nor sweeter milk can help.

Tasteless and odourless, it is left to skin in reproach. Some unnamed respiratory virus has made those two inseparables, smell and taste, gang up on me.

As I hurry through my kitchen chores every morning, I revel in the scents that swirl about me. They waft me to destinations unexplored or to the comforting spaces of childhood, and rescue me from the banalities of the moment.

When I crush a plump clove of garlic to emancipate its lilting signature of odours and smell nothing, I sniff vigorously to clear my nose. And then, with the schnozz clear as a whistle, if I still can't smell the garlic, I should be seriously worried.

One of the earliest symptoms of Covid-19 is the loss of smell and taste.

When you don't have a stuffy nose and yet can't smell garlic, it startles you. As it startled nearly 60 per cent of Covid-19 patients, who reported anosmia, loss of smell, and dysgeusia, loss of taste.

The nasal and oral cavities are traps for two of life's greatest pleasures, smell and taste. Their soft, moist lining has trillions of special sensors to inform and warn us of coming dangers or pleasures. Without this information, we would be clueless—not just about gastronomy but about our neighbours too. It is not polite to mention it, but every person has a distinctive aroma that battles past barriers of scented soap and deodorants to assert itself as identity.

Without smell and taste, it is a dull world.

And, it might be dangerous too.

Are these trillions of smell and taste receptors receptacles for SARS-CoV-2? ACE2 is liberally sprinkled on this velvety lining of the nose and mouth. Is it the honey trap?

Atop the nasal cavity and separated from its turbulence by the *lamina cribrosa,* a perforated wafer of bone, thinner than a potato chip, rests the brain. Scary, isn't it, the brain being so close to the exterior?

This exposed bit of the brain has to do with smell. The olfactory bulbs snuggled beneath the cerebrum receive and process information from the olfactory epithelium, the 'smelling' fringe of the nose. The olfactory epithelium is so full of nerves, it is almost a layer of brain. These nerves pierce the bone chip and relay smells to the olfactory bulbs.

The upper airway is rich in ACE2 receptors—so densely present that it may well be a viral reservoir. Does this viral reservoir include the nerve cells of smell? If so, it is a shortcut for the virus to enter the brain. Now that is a terrifying thought.

Animal studies suggest a reassuring fact: it is the *other* cells of the olfactory epithelium, not the neurons, that express ACE2. Anosmia, the earliest sign of impending Covid-19, may be the result of inflammation in these cells. Inflammatory factors may either directly impact the neuronal cells or dampen their signalling. The olfactory bulbs would then have information blackout, and one might walk past a rose with a perfunctory nod to its colour, but otherwise unmoved.

Reassuringly, most patients recover their sense of smell. And may they savour every molecule of life—bon appétit!

But there still remains that scary thought of the brain being just a sneeze away. Can Covid-19 affect the brain?

Many 'neurological symptoms' have been reported in large patient series from Wuhan and elsewhere. People have experienced a spectrum of worrying aliments, from dizziness and tics to full-blown strokes. It is not uncommon to find these problems cropping up in any major illness, and these people have been severely ill. The question is: are these nervous illnesses part of the general profile and its complications, or does the virus specifically target nervous tissue?

That's a very apposite question.

The brain has its own immune system and is protected from the general chaos of the rest of the body by a magical membrane, the blood–brain barrier. Infections that involve the brain occur when this barrier is breached, either by pathogens themselves or by the cells and chemicals of the immune response. Does this happen in Covid-19?

Does SARS-CoV-2 specifically target the nervous system? The term for such a virus is 'neurotropic'. Two well known illnesses caused by neurotropic viruses are polio and rabies.

Neurological symptoms are more common in severe Covid-19 cases. In patients who died, changes in the brain have been noted at autopsy.

The cerebrospinal fluid (CSF) is a nourishing and protective fluid that circulates around the brain and spinal cord. It is separated from the bloodstream by membranes. Viral particles have been found from the CSF of severely ill patients.

Recently, a New York facility reported strokes in young patients with early lung signs of Covid-19. Also noticed, sporadically, in Covid-19 patients is the Guillain-Barré syndrome, a transient paralysis which sets in as an autoimmune reaction after recovery from the initial infection. SARS and MERS, the two earlier infections with coronaviruses, also showed central nervous system changes in severely affected patients.

There are multiple ways in which SARS-CoV-2 can enter the sacred spaces of the brain and spinal cord. And there are ways in which it can target this delicate tissue simply through its effects on immunity.

3. Poisoned!

The commonest worry people voice is: *Can food and water be infected by this virus?* Poisoning is the ultimate human terror, after all. Treachery in the wellsprings of life is an unendurable thought, but it is also an uncontrollable disaster. Considering which, isn't it remarkable how complacently we've been eating food poisoned with pesticides, drinking water loaded with dioxins and breathing air choked with pollutants for years now?

Of course, the virus can and will be shed in saliva and stool. That should have been self-evident once we learnt what its receptor was. The question is, how long will it stay viable and infectious once it is shed?

Meanwhile, many patients have experienced 'stomach problems' as their first evidence of illness. While this is anecdotal, a Stanford investigation of 116 patients with respiratory symptoms showed a high incidence of dyspepsia and liver functions. On examining the spectrum of gastrointestinal complaints in COVID-19 patients, they seem to stretch from oesophageal to colonic. So where is the virus sequestered in the gastrointestinal tract?

Can SARS-CoV-2 selectively infect the gastrointestinal tract?

Where in the miles of intestine is there a situation comparable to the airway?

Everywhere.

There are ACE2 receptors all along the length of the digestive tract. Also present is the cellular serine protease, or transmembrane protease serine 2 (TMPRSS2), that cleaves the spike protein of human coronaviruses on the cell membrane. Since both systems of cell entry are present, it is not unexpected that SARS-CoV-2 should engage with them. But how on earth does the virus get past stomach acid? There may be a different route of viral entry to the digestive tract.

4. Heartache

People with heart and blood vessel disease have a bad Covid-19 profile. Their numbers are high in the ARDS group, which means many of them die. Considering cardiovascular disease is the planet's number one killer, this is a very worrying observation. In 2017, 17.8 million people died of cardiovascular disease and more than three-fourths of this number were from middle- and low-income countries. That means a very large number of people at very high risk for ARDS, should they suffer from Covid-19.

Why are they so susceptible?

The answer came to us circumspectly, from other body organs usually ignored in the Covid-19 reckoning. Seriously ill Covid-19 patients, already in respiratory failure, often develop crises in other body organs: kidney shutdown, intestinal infarction, liver failure. These affected organs—some post-mortem, some in surgically removed tissue—reveal a common denominator. In diverse organs, with diverse pathologies, the target tissue is the same: *the inner lining of blood vessels, the endothelium.*

The endothelium is much more than inner-wear. It is responsible for regulating a number of vascular functions, from blood pressure to laminar blood flow. It maintains the cardiovascular system in a state of health and preparedness. When the endothelium is sick, blood vessels constrict to cause a slew of troubles. Narrowed vessels means less blood supply. Organs deprived of oxygen react with oedema and switch to a pro-coagulatory state. This worsens as oxygen-starved cells die, either in small clusters or across a swathe of tissue, causing organ shutdown. The blood now has micro-thrombi, tiny clots, as the clotting mechanism goes haywire. In Covid-19, the endothelium is stuffed with migrant inflammatory cells, and the endothelial cells themselves are heavily laden with SARS-CoV-2 particles.

This is evidence enough that SARS-CoV-2 targets the endothelium—which is rich in ACE2 receptors—early in the disease. Covid-19 is a multi-organ menace.

The heart is also a target. Cardiac muscle cells show signs of injury. This may be part of the generalised cytokine storm or a direct effect of the virus. The frightening cardiac effects of Covid-19 simply tell us that we have been irresponsible in ignoring the leading cause of mortality: cardiovascular disease.

5. Covid Junior

For three months into Covid-19, it was assumed that children were safe from the virus.

By early April, that complacence was painfully dented, urging hindsight. A revised view stated that children were just as likely to catch the virus, but less likely to experience the worst from the disease. Then, mid-April, the South Thames Retrieval Service in London, which provides care for 2 million children, noted a cluster of ten children who presented with a shock syndrome, rather like what is encountered in Kawasaki disease.[9]

The children had been well when they were struck by fever, rash, conjunctivitis and diarrhoea. This progressed quickly to shock, and required critical care. None of

9. Dr Tomisaku Kawasaki died on 5 June 2020 in Tokyo. He was 95. In 1967, he described what he called 'mucocutaneous lymph node syndrome', an occasionally fatal acquired heart disease in children.

them had ARDS. None tested positive for viral particles in respiratory secretions. After discharge from hospital, two children tested positive. The overall picture was that of multi-organ involvement, with heart muscle and blood vessel damage. These children had been in contact with COVID-19-positive family members. The alert sounded by these observations led to more cases being reported.

In the United States, by April, many children, similarly afflicted, were rushed to hospital, many with cardiac symptoms. The condition was labelled hyper-inflammatory syndrome, for want of a better name. It is now called Childhood Multi-System Inflammatory Syndrome, or MIS-C. Many of these children are not COVID-positive on PCR, but they do have antibodies suggesting a recent infection.

This is a frightening new manifestation of COVID-19. Some paediatricians feel it should more properly be regarded as a sequel to the infection.

And, once again, the culprit is inflammation.

6. COVID Next Gen

The most horrendous fallout of any infection is injury to mother and foetus during pregnancy. It is the sad lot of paediatric surgeons to focus on this segment of disease. Of the many congenital anomalies (read birth defects) we encounter, the worst are the category of 'foetal disruptions', an aggregate of complications that involve all the major body organs. Babies with these are born with visible 'deformities' that are soon evident as disorders of function, many life-threatening; a baby with a cleft lip and palate may have structural defects in the brain, kidneys, spine, heart and intestines too.

TORCH stands for common pathogens that cause such injuries to the foetus:

Toxoplasma,
Rubella,
Cytomegalovirus and
Herpes.

O now stands for 'Other', an expansile catch-as-catch-can term for every emerging disease.

We saw foetal disruption happen with Zika virus in the worst possible way.

Could it happen with COVID-19?

When a maternal infection crosses the placenta and enters foetal circulation, it can impact the developing organs of the baby. Infection depends on the severity of maternal infection, on the virulence of the virus and the immune response. This last is always a vexed field in pregnancy. Potentially, sperm is a threat to the mother's body as it is 'non-self'. By extension, so is the embryo. A state of immune tolerance is quickly established, and the embryo is nurtured as the most important of a mother's organs. The foetus becomes her physiological priority, overriding all the demands of her own body.

Pregnancy is one of the greatest wonders of nature, and science hasn't yet discovered the half of it.

If a pathogen is virulent enough to cross the placenta but not virulent enough to kill the foetus, pregnancy continues, with tragic results. The actively dividing cells of the early embryo are viral targets. Viruses impact the formation of body organs, and this results in defects in structures concealed within the body's cavities. Since the body's exterior development is paced by what it protects, the development of the exterior, too, doesn't proceed along expected lines and many babies so affected will be born looking 'different'. For example, Zika virus attacks the developing brain. The development of the skull is dictated by the development of the brain. When the afflicted foetal brain fails to achieve its expected size, so does the skull. Babies with congenital Zika syndrome are born with microcephaly—posh for a small head.

When a pathogen affects the embryo, it will attack all vulnerable organs, impacting them in their prevailing phase of development. Such babies may be born with a bewildering array of seemingly random deformities. But they are all linked by the common denominator of foetal insult.

The *timing* of maternal infection is all important.

Infections in the first trimester, when foetal organs are in the process of being formed, can result in structural defects, very often visible on ultrasound a little further into pregnancy. If the infection is overwhelming, the foetus cannot survive. Maternal infections later in pregnancy affect foetal growth or overwhelm the foetus with direct injury or toxemia.

The foetus is a target in all maternal infections.

Will SARS-CoV-2 attack the foetus?

What will Covid-19 in a pregnant woman do to her baby?

So far, we don't know much. There are accounts of successful deliveries of normal babies by women who suffered from Covid-19 in the last trimester. This is heartening but not informative enough.

We want to know how Covid-19 can impact foetal development.

Can it cross the placenta?

Does the placenta have ACE2 receptors?

Does the foetus?

Does SARS-CoV-2 have a particular tissue target? (Zika virus, for instance, is neurotropic, and it latches on to developing nervous tissue.)

An early series from Wuhan, of 118 pregnant women who had COVID-19, is optimistic. There were seventy births during the study period. The babies tested negative. Some mothers became sicker after delivery but eventually recovered. Samples of breast milk were clear of virus particles.

These women were infected late in pregnancy. The impact expected on the foetus is growth-related, but there was no such growth retardation. Neither were the babies born with respiratory symptoms. They didn't progress to the dreaded respiratory distress syndrome (the paediatric version of ARDS).

This could be interpreted as evidence that the virus does not cross the placental barrier.

More recent reports aren't so complacent. At this point, case reports are more than anecdotes, and here's one from the third week of February 2020, from Renmin Hospital, Wuhan, China:

On 28 January, a woman of twenty-nine was diagnosed with COVID-19. She was thirty-four weeks pregnant. Her lungs had the typical changes associated with the disease on CT scan. She was in respiratory distress. The virus was isolated from her nasopharyngeal secretions. She was hospitalised on 2 February and treated with antibiotics, antivirals and steroids. On 21 February, tests showed she had circulating antibodies to COVID-19, both immunoglobulin G (IgG) and immunoglobulin M (IgM). On 22 February, she delivered a daughter by caesarean section. A poignant line in the report reads: *The mother wore an N95 mask and did not hold the infant.*

The baby was healthy but underwent repeated nasopharyngeal swab testing from the age of two hours to sixteen days. Though the test was consistently negative, her blood showed signs of having undergone SARS-CoV-2 infection. Antibodies, both IgG and IgM, were present. CT scans of her lungs were clear.

The mother recuperated. Her breast milk did not show any viral particles.

This case report is an eye-opener. The baby's antibodies tell us that she was infected too. IgG is the usual maternal antibody found in the newborn, but IgM is too large a molecule to cross the placenta. The foetus begins manufacturing IgM from the twentieth week of intrauterine life, and this one responded to the virus in her circulation with a protective surge of antibody.

This case report appeared on 26 March and jolted the world out of its earlier complacence about pregnancies in COVID-19. Earlier reports had no evidence of the virus having affected the baby, despite extensive testing.

What routes of infection can carry SARS-CoV-2 into the baby?

a. Trans-placental is the greatest worry. Evidence from babies born through caesarean section suggest this is possible.

b. From the mother's vaginal canal and perineum, during delivery. We do know that the virus is shed in the faeces, and such contamination is possible during labour.

c. Through breast milk. This is of utmost importance, and there's very little data on this so far.

Do other coronaviruses affect the foetus?

Experiments on animals infected with appropriate coronaviruses (MCoVirus, which affects mice) have produced infected offspring. Pregnant cats suffering from coronavirus feline peritonitis give birth to infected kittens.

Data from 100 pregnant women who were infected by SARS-CoV in the 2003 epidemic has been analysed: nothing suggests this virus ever infected the foetus.

Months into this epidemic, we're still unclear about a vital question. Will COVID-19 affect the next generation?

Judging from the conflicting reports, it's too early to tell if safe pregnancy is possible in a COVID-positive woman. It does seem wiser not to risk it.

Strangely, there are no reports so far of the vaginal lining having been tested for viral particles. An omission, as the vagina is in direct communication with the pelvic cavity, and if infected, can be a route to serious abdominal disease. In pregnant women, a vaginal infection can be a route to the foetus. And of course it will also mean COVID-19 can be sexually transmitted. There is no news of this yet, and we need to know.

The male reproductive tract is by no means safe from the virus. In a study of thirty-eight semen samples collected from men in different stages of COVID-19, viral particles were found in six patients. Four of them were on the critical list, but the other two were recovering. It's important to know how long the viral particles persisted.

The persistence of a virus does not necessarily mean active disease, but are such viral particles infectious?

What about sex? Can SARS-CoV-2 be transmitted between partners? Certainly, such proximity means breathing each other's exhalations. And the virus is likely to be shared by more routes than one.

So, what is safe sex in the time of COVID-19? Masked and gloved?

Whatever.

Just don't wear a condom on your heart.

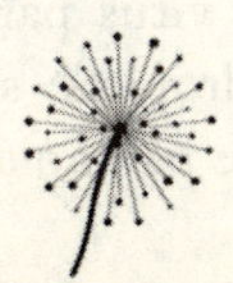

24
Viral Shedding

> We seek him here, we seek him there,
> Those Frenchies seek him everywhere.
> Is he in heaven?—Is he in hell?
> That demmed, elusive Pimpernel.
>
> – Baroness Emmuska Orczy, *The Scarlet Pimpernel*, 1905

Where does SARS-CoV-2 lurk?

The gimlet eyes of masked passers-by suggest I radiate the virus from every pore. Do I?

I'm flooded with offers to disinfect my home, my possessions, my building with WHO-approved chemicals, and who's to argue against such aegis?

I can now buy milk 'untouched by hand'. From udder to udhar, so to say. But I was knocked cold by a similar offer of vegetables, tubers included. I tried to imagine the safe transit of nature's bounty, guaranteed virus-free.

It simply cannot be done.

In all the objects that compose our tactile world, where does SARS-CoV-2 lurk?

Lurk is insulting. The virus is simply living out its destiny.

But where?

Within us, on us, everywhere.

Saliva, nasal drips and air, coughed out or exhaled by infected people, contain virus particles. The virus is shot out in a fine spray of droplets; scary animations abound for the credulous and the paranoid. As though this weren't enough, we now learn that our exhalations are propelled on a turbulent cloud of moist air that keeps the virus aloft for a greater time and distance than we believed. Six feet may be an underestimation of how far those droplets travel before they settle—where?

On surfaces all around us. Surfaces we touch. And, in panic, disinfect.

How logical is this?

Viruses cannot exist outside a host cell. The aerosol an infected person sneezes, coughs, speaks or, simply, exhales is a mixture of infected cells and a crowd of organic molecules from respiratory secretions in a fog of humidity. How long does the virus survive in this aerosol?

Low relative humidity and cold temperatures keep enveloped viruses viable for longer. Larger particles settle quicker, and the size of the infecting particle depends on both virus size and the organic matter to which it is attached. That explains why viruses last longer in the air of clean scrubbed surroundings than they do in filthy areas, which contain larger particles in suspension.

So, the size of the suspended particle is what decides the infectivity. Larger particles are likely to settle quickly. And if inhaled, will be pushed out by the cilia. Smaller particles stay suspended in the air for longer durations and get past the cilia when inhaled.

It is optimistic, and futile, to imagine that viral transmission can be restricted to a limited space.

The survival times of viral particles on surfaces has been clocked: x hours for plastic, y for metal, z for clothing, and so on. Thankfully, this is being eased up to a more logical attitude. The virus may not be so easily transmitted from surfaces after all.

What does count is the population density, the crowd factor.

The lockdown is an extreme example of reducing the number of people per square foot of public space. It ignores the realities of poor countries like India, Brazil, Ecuador, and most of Asia and Africa, where restricting the occupation of public spaces means intense overcrowding of private spaces—homes, corridors, staircases, shelters. A large proportion of the populace in these countries are the homeless or migrants, thousands of miles away from home. No epidemiological prediction can have any meaning if they are ignored.

Disease is not a political landscape, it is an intimately personal one. Whatever government policy may be, it is our own immediate policy of behaviour that will keep us healthy.

SARS-CoV-2 is shed maximally in the early phase of infection. So it is safe policy to have some degree of barrier between the home and the street.

~ Changing your footwear, washing your hands and other exposed areas on entering the house.

~ Maintaining a physical distance of six to ten feet from your neighbours in a public space.

~ Wearing a clean mask in public spaces, where mandatory. (Wash daily if yours is a homemade cloth mask.)

~ Avoiding public gatherings.

These measures should be sufficient. Disinfection with soap and water is ample.

Disinfectants are an entire new can of worms. The post-COVID-19 world will be full of resistant bacteria. Mysterious hormonal and neurological diseases will emerge as consequence of our eagerness to rely on chemical cleansers. Bleach, used in a suitable dilution, is effective for cleaning large spaces or spills of bodily secretions. But it is a dangerous idea to spray it. The fog will stay suspended for a while. Inhaling it can spell disaster to the Covid-threatened lung.

What of body secretions?

~ The Churchillian blood, sweat and tears, plus saliva, nasal drip and coughed out phlegm, can all infect.

~ Semen carries virus particles for several weeks after infection, but there is no proof that it is infective. Nothing, as yet, is definite about the sexual transmission of this disease.

~ The urine of infected patients occasionally carries virus particles. But is it infective?

~ The gastrointestinal tract is a virus hideout for sure. From oesophagus to colon, it is well supplied with ACE2 receptors for the virus to engage with. No surprise, then, that diarrhoea is often a presenting symptom of Covid-19. It is to be expected that the stools should contain shed virus.

Viral shedding in stools continues for at least a week beyond the persistence of viral particles in saliva and snot. Spread through stools—elegantly put, faecal–oral contamination—is common with many viruses. Besides those that cause gastroenteritis, hepatitis A & E and poliovirus spread thus. So does SARS-CoV-2.

Sewage has been studied for viral load by estimating virus particles in raw sludge. The number of cases in a community correlates unmistakably with the viral load in sewage. This means sewage viral load can be used as a reliable predictor of an outbreak. It can be an effective tool for viral surveillance.

Faecal–oral transmission, by the way, is as common in populations that have regular sanitation and running water as it is in poorer countries with no sanitation worth the mention. Having facilities is one thing—using them, quite another.

Looking at the pre-COVID-19 era, which feels like Deep Time these days, I am taken back to the last film I saw in Manhattan. Joaquin Phoenix's *Joker* was wiped clean from my memory by what I observed in the packed restroom. As relieved New Yorkers emerged from their cubicles, not one stopped by the washbasins. The toilet paper crisis, so loudly bewailed, might be a godsend. Washing more than hands will be a significant step in limiting the spread of COVID-19.

India's Swachh Bharat Abhiyan, or Clean India Mission, has not assured hygienic, usable indoor toilets while militating aggressively against open-air defecation. In incidents so shaming that they don't bear writing about, vigilantes have beaten, tortured and killed people caught defecating in the open. Cruelty cannot sink lower than this.

Once more, a disease challenges us.

Do we respond with hate or with sapience?

My steepled hands in anjali mudra connect my heart with yours, as I wish you namaste. Like the eastern etiquette of bowing, this form of greeting may have begun as a precaution against contagion by faecal-oral transmission. Around the time this became rife, other cultures familiar to India shook hands instead.

The oldest known record of a handshake is an Assyrian bas relief from the ninth century BCE. In the limestone photo-op, the Assyrian king Shalmaneser III and the Babylonian king Marduk-zakir-shumi I shake hands.

Whether in greeting, alliance or reconciliation, we can no longer tell, but it is an unmistakable gesture of solidarity.

Perhaps the namaste displaced the handshake 5,000 years ago for much the same reason as it has in this time of Covid-19.

All the more reason to appreciate the thought behind it: *From my heart, to yours…*

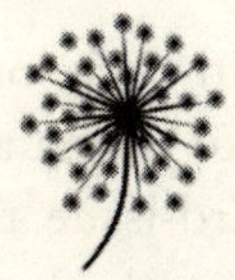

25
Elsewhere, Everywhere

I, like an usurp'd town to another due,
Labor to admit you, but oh, to no end;
– John Donne, *Holy Sonnet XIV*, 1609

The ubiquity of ACE2 in body organs is well established. We still need to get used to the truth that the body has more 'organs' than the standard-issue textbook picture tells us. Skin is one of the most overlooked organs. So is fat.

Fat is much more than the bulge we battle. It is an organised tissue, a hormone factory closely linked to and deeply influenced by the gut microbiome. The equatorial bulge that makes a snazzy T-shirt intemperately snug isn't wardrobe dysfunction, it is body dysfunction. It is a disease called obesity.

For years now, the relationship between fat and the metabolic syndrome has been well recognised. Metabolic syndrome is a convenient label for the triad of obesity, high blood pressure and dyslipidemia, evident on blood tests as an abnormal lipid profile. Metabolic syndrome is a pre-diabetic condition that, if left untreated, will lead to diabetes and cardiovascular disease.

For most obese people, being overweight is not an illness, it is a cosmetic problem. Nevertheless, after complications appear, obesity becomes more than an inconvenient dress size. What are these complications?

Diabetes.

High blood pressure and other cardiovascular diseases.

Liver and kidney diseases.

Arthritis.
Infertility.
And, Covid-19?

Covid-19 causes early, often severe, complications in the obese. It is one of the most worrying observations of late, and we cannot afford to ignore it. It is particularly crucial because many of those unfortunate victims are very young.

Obesity is the pandemic we have chosen to ignore. In some countries, obesity affects over 40 per cent of the population. In others, it is as low as 5 per cent.

It is the poorer, more disadvantaged, nations that have a growing obese population. Especially among the young, Asian standards of obesity are very different from the Western norm. Asians are more liable to develop complications, specifically heart disease, very early into obesity.

A BMI of 23 is edging overweight for an Indian, but is quite within limits for an American. The BMI itself is a vexed index. All of which bears out my deep mistrust in statistics.

If you want to find out how common obesity is, take a walk and count the paunches that stride past you.

You'll find few on a quiet street. But a saunter past the railway or bus station will get you many more. And if you really want numbers, go into a school yard at lunch time; childhood obesity is a nightmare.

Obesity is fat. Slabs and slabs of it. Beneath the skin and within body cavities, visible and deeply concealed, it builds up at the cost of other body tissue.

Don't, even for a moment, mistake fat for a chunk of mindless grease. Fat is made up of adipocytes, some of the most intelligent and wired cells in the body.

Fat fascinates me enough to occupy a lot of my thinking time, but right now, the one aspect of the adipocyte I worry about is its role in the renin-angiotensin system.

Why would fat have a say in the renin-angiotensin system?

Well, fat takes up a lot of body space, and therefore, it must have miles of blood vessels looping about to keep it nourished, and the renin-angiotensin system is all about maintaining blood pressure, right?

Sure. That's the thought we broke our teeth on fifty years ago.

But in the light of recent discoveries, we know that fat probably regulates and controls this axis. Being so widely distributed throughout the body, how can fat *not* have a say in inflammation?

We know now that fat is vociferous in its contribution to inflammation. Fat deposits—white adipose tissue—are high in ACE, with its strong pro-inflammatory cellular and chemical profile. As fat deposits increase, so does ACE. Pro-inflammatory, ACE-stimulated cytokines secreted locally in fat deposits have far-reaching effects. They enter the circulation and set up a generalised state of chronic inflammation, which affects every organ of the body. The metabolic effects of obesity—diabetes, abnormal circulating fats, fatty deposition in the liver, atherosclerosis—are soon seen.

How does obesity change the dynamics of Covid-19?

It seems to make younger patients susceptible to dire complications. Increased inflammatory factors are noticed early in the disease, cardiac damage is common, and the disordered blood clotting that heralds multi-organ failure soon sets in.

The link between obesity and ARDS is not unexpected, as it has been noticed in earlier epidemics of viral pneumonia, during both the H1N1 flu epidemic of 2009 and the SARS epidemic of 2003. The enhanced inflammatory profile in obese patients was noticed then. We overlooked or forgot that warning, and ignored the link between obesity and ARDS in Covid-19. We cannot afford to do so any longer.

Obesity must be treated, not left to 'try and reduce' advice. Right now, this is a matter of some urgency.

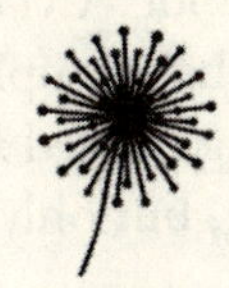

26
Silica, Silica

L'illusion est le premier plaisir.

– Voltaire, *La Pucella d'Orleans*, 1756

22 April 2020. The reports crowding this fourth month of the pandemic are not about ARDS. A sort of resolution has been arrived at over that complication. More and more, pneumonias are now being treated *without* ventilator therapy. The results are promising, but only cohort analysis will tell, and that will take a while.

This week's concerns are about multi-organ involvement or failure. Kidneys shut down, hearts fail, patients slip into coma or wake up to find themselves paralysed.

Headlines like *'What Does COVID-19 Do to Your Brain?'; 'COVID-19 Patients Can Die of Kidney Failure'; 'COVID-19 Damages the Heart' and 'Neuropsychiatric Complications of COVID-19'* warn of greater terrors that lie in wait.

Or not.

These communiqués unleash all the horrors clinicians are trained to anticipate from the developing profile of any serious illness. Each organ functions as a signpost. Each new manifestation is a punctuation in the breathless narrative of overwhelming disease. For the physician it is a near-ritualistic pause.

This moment of doubt and introspection and, yes, of terror, summons up hidden reserves of skill and understanding. And this is very evident in the analyses of these complications that clinicians and pathologists have published, many as pre-print articles, to urgently share their insights.

Again, this reveals the dichotomy in our perception. The news is weighted on the villainy of the virus, projected as all the demons of myth and memory rolled into one. Reality, on the other hand, is weighted on human suffering, the body's own destructive response to the virus.

There are no barricades that will keep any virus out of our lives. SARS-CoV-2 cannot be, will not be, contained either by isolation or by lockdown. As testing becomes more easily available, and hopefully reliable, we may discover that almost everyone tests positive. Herd immunity, the evidence that we've all grown resistant to the virus, hasn't shown itself yet. This should tell us that the only way out of this mess is to focus on the body's own response. And that is exactly what researchers are working on as we move closer to new, intelligent therapies.

Meanwhile, the body doesn't exist in a vacuum, even during lockdowns. So, how is our external milieu shaping this pandemic?

Today is Earth Day—the fiftieth, in fact. Like doctors who ask for tests before they examine a patient, we can review the earth's indices in terms of climate change: albedo, air quality indices, carbon sink, greenhouse gases, glacier dissolutions, Milankovich variations, nephology. The list is unending.

Or, we could simply look out of the window.

What do you see when you do?

No matter where you live, you probably will see—on a clear day—a blue sky. A sky bluer than the one you were used to.

Since the outbreak of Covid-19, vehicle emissions have gone down, factories have closed, air travel has plummeted, our crowds and activity have thinned.

Return to that cold December morning in Wuhan and

once more join our three friends awaiting medical attention.

The air Guan-Yin, Jiān and Bohai had been exposed to was very different—filled with a heavy burden of particulate matter. Over the past decade, Wuhan has been transformed into an impressive city of towering buildings, a frenzy that has involved the transfer of stone, marble, cement, concrete and sand. In whatever form, sourced no matter wherefrom, bits of these building materials have been wafted by the wind as particles of silica, silicon dioxide.

Silicon dioxide has a very long and fraught history with our lungs. We have breathed it since—perhaps even before—we were human. Silicon dioxide makes up 60 per cent of the earth's crust. More significantly, it answers a basic human need that often even supersedes our imperatives of food and sex.

Silica is beautiful; it invites self-expression. As stone, as gem, as pigment, silica is a treasury of light, colour and texture. Our ancestors simply couldn't resist it, and neither can we. We paint with it, we sculpt with it, we build with it, we wear it and we hoard it. And, all the time, we breathe it.

Our lungs have had a continuous exposure to silica of different grades for 50,000 years.

Two years ago, my puzzling observations on Dholavira led me to investigate this fraught relationship, and I didn't have to look far to find a population that practically mirrored the vanished past.

The city of Khambat has a long memory of the agate trade, clearly documented at least since the tenth century CE. Today it is struggling to keep the trade going. The reason? Agate workers, inheritors of the ancient skills of cutting and polishing, are dying of silicosis.

And it isn't just agate workers who are plagued by inhaled silica.

In a country like India, where industrial giants are powered by unorganised labour, the victim of silicosis is ignored, easily expendable, and rapidly replaced. Entire villages and communities of stoneworkers have been impoverished, often annihilated, by silicosis.

Not just India. China has a very high incidence of silicosis. As has Iran. As has Italy. As, probably, does the rest of the world.

Silicosis is the best kept secret of capitalism. The number of victims through human memory is staggering, but at least history notices them. Their stories have been recorded over the centuries.

Today's victims are less fortunate.

Silicosis, the disease, may be limited to those with a prolonged and intensive exposure to such factories and mines. But all of us are exposed to silica as inhaled dust. The commonest source in burgeoning cities is the building boom and upscale home remodelling, a thriving and unceasing cottage industry.

Particulates in the air with a diameter below 2.5 micrometres—about 3 per cent of the diameter of a human hair—are specified as PM2.5. They are the size that sneaks past the cleaning crew in the airway and reaches the alveoli. Bigger particles are not innocuous either. The constant irritation of the upper airways they cause is associated with nasopharyngeal cancers, which are well documented in stone workers.

Fine silica particles set up a reaction that leads to the disease called silicosis.[10] In its long-standing form, silicosis

---

10. One of the longest words in the dictionary, *supercalifragilisticexpialidocious*, loses out to a cousin of silicosis, *pneumonoultramicroscopicsilicovolcanocosis*—the lung disease caused by ultramicroscopic silica dust derived from volcanic eruptions.

is debilitating, as it slowly but inexorably chokes off respiratory reserves. Victims begin with a nagging cough that progresses to wheezing and breathlessness. Often, tuberculosis or other bacterial infections supervene and hurtle the victim into crisis. Most pathetic of all is acute silicosis, a disease which destroys within days, ending in ARDS, a picture very like the terminal phase of Covid-19.

What is happening within the lung in silicosis? Once you start examining that picture, it is almost impossible to look away. Like the *Panchatantra,* which has stories scrolled tight within stories, or like a painting by Hieronymus Bosch, crowded with unfinished incident, the lung-scape of silicosis is both urgent and leisurely, so I'll merely pause at a few signposts here:

The first cell that responds to the presence of silica in the alveolus is the type 2 alveolar cell, which responds with a surge in the production of surfactant. This secretion coats the silica particle to reduce its toxicity temporarily. But that's of questionable benefit: surfactant overproduction causes lung injury.

The coated silica is taken up by the most important player in silicosis, the alveolar macrophage. It has surface receptors that engage with silica, the most important of these being MARCO (macrophage receptor with collagenous structure). The entry of silica into the cell sets off a series of toxic reactions that end with apoptosis.

The internalisation of silica also releases free radicals, reactive oxygen species (ROS) and reactive nitrogen species (RNS). Freshly fractured silica has a greater potential for free-radical generation. Free radicals are cell killers, and cause lung injury at many levels by turning on cellular pathways that initiate the inflammation cascade.

Meanwhile, the internalised particles are stored in a vesicle (lysosome) and drenched with digestive enzymes, all in vain. The macrophage cannot digest silica. The lysosome begins to leak and sets off reactions that lead to cell death. Excessive cell death induces, very soon, an autoimmune state. Victims of silicosis suffer from a variety of autoimmune disorders.

The lung's ultimate fate is fibrosis—the apoptosed, dead macrophages set off chronic inflammation, and fibrosis develops around the extruded particles of silica.

Also of note is the observation that the alveolar macrophages that engulf silica consume a lot of fat (lipids), giving them a 'foamy' appearance under the microscope. The type of fat that 'foams' the silicotic alveolar macrophages is Ox-LDL, an oxidised variant of the circulating low-density lipoprotein (LDL). Unlike its unoxidised form, Ox-LDL promotes cellular dysfunction by activating inflammatory pathways. It also triggers fibrotic change.

Silica-exposed lungs are, therefore, in a state of chronic inflammation. When SARS-CoV-2 engages the ACE2 receptors in the type 2 alveolar cells, the innate immune response is unbridled and aggressive, causing diffuse alveolar destruction. The patient records this change by becoming increasingly breathless, and by entering into the end state of ARDS.

Wuhan has had a fraught AQI. It is in this setting that Guan-Yin, Jiān and Bohai inhaled that silent sinister dose of SARS-CoV-2.

Is there a nexus between inhaled particulates, particularly silica, and the devastating picture of Covid-19?

I think there is. China has a very high incidence of silicosis. Silica sources are legion. I prefer to look at silica as one of the PM2.5 pollutants inhaled in ambient air by the general population.

In January 2013, all of China's megacities suffered severe haze pollution, with the daily PM2.5 concentration peaking at 772 μg m^3.[11] Wuhan is an expanding centre of rapid urbanisation, with a population of over 10 million. In a two-year study, the daily PM2.5 concentrations ranged between 106.5–114.9 μg m^3. While local sources were aplenty, Wuhan also received a great deal of particulate matter from adjoining regions. December 2013 was the haziest month in Wuhan, attributed to increased local emissions, low temperature, low wind speed and high pressure. Particulate matter showed two diurnal peaks, coinciding with traffic emissions. The haze formation in Wuhan originated from the provinces north and south of Wuhan—Baoding and Handan in Hebei province, Zhumadian in Henan province, Bozhou in Anhui province, Xiaoyi in Shanxi province, Taian in Shandong province and Changsha in Hunan province.

The ambient air in December 2019 couldn't have been very different.

In any respiratory illness, air quality is vital to recovery. We know this from the household measures we use while treating coughs and colds.

Following the outbreak of COVID-19, the containment measures in Wuhan brought the city to a standstill.

One of the immediate effects was clear skies.

As the haze lifted, the PM2.5 levels plummeted.

When the epidemic folded up, it was attributed to the draconian isolation measures clamped on the city.

I have a contrarian view.

I think the coincidental reduction in PM2.5 particulates reduced airway irritation. The inflammatory balance in the

11. The concentration of an air pollutant is measured in micrograms (one-millionth of a gram) per cubic metre air or μg/m^3.

lung was restored. Now, when the same virus was inhaled, innate immunity worked efficiently. Milder symptoms and recovery followed. A large part of the population remained asymptomatic. ARDS stopped.

In months to come, we may hear more from brilliant Chinese scientists on the nexus between particulate matter and SARS-CoV-2. And I may be proved wrong in my surmise.

However, three facts are indisputable:

~ Silica injures the lungs and leaves them in a state of chronic inflammation.

~ Most of us living in crowded cities inhale highly polluted air on a daily basis, of which silica PM2.5 is a key component.

~ This makes the lungs vulnerable to uncontrollable inflammation—not just from COVID-19 but from every other respiratory pathogen out there already or slouching towards Bethlehem to emerge.

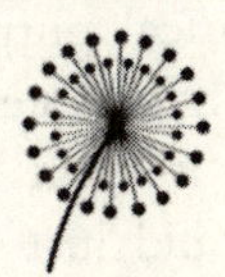

27
The Book of the Dead

True journey is return.

– Ursula K. Le Guin, *The Dispossessed: An Ambiguous Utopia*, 1974

The Egyptian 'Book of the Dead' was never called that by the Egyptians. The tag is a translation of the naïve and very literal descriptive grave robbers in the nineteenth century gave the papyri they found buried with mummiya.[12] *Kitāb al Maiyytun* had enough mystique for the Victorian Egyptologist to know he was on to a good thing, and so the *Book of the Dead* it became. The Egyptians who wrote the papyri had a more resonant title: 'Coming Forth into the Day'. The spells the text contained promised to 'make his soul flourish, and prevent him from dying the (second) death'.

Doctors everywhere read the Book of the Dead for this very purpose. We read the dead to prevent a second death. That has been the historical purpose of autopsy, though pre-historically, it may have been compelled by simple curiosity. We arrogantly imagine our ancestors as jejune hunter-gatherers, who could just about brain an antelope and grill a steak. But they also made kitchen knives you can use today, jewellery that makes Cartier look rustic and art that would send Picasso sulking back into his Blue Period. And we humans were surgeons before we became hunter-gatherers. Injuries had to heal, babies had to be birthed, and it required skill to do all that. When those skills failed,

---

12. From early medieval times, European medicine had relied on mummia as the secret ingredient in elixirs, but the trade really hotted up in the nineteenth century. The word 'mummy' is a corruption of 'mom' for bitumen, used to preserve the dead in ancient Egypt.

surely the surgeon wanted to know why. So she, or maybe he, looked inside to discover what had stilled the body's exuberance. The dead body was the first textbook.

Death transforms the profane body into sacred space through the chemistry of decay. Disgust quickly becomes dread, and taboo is but a word away. Colluded unhappily with the afterlife, death is closed to further enquiry.

Opening the Book of the Dead is as difficult today as it was in Europe during the Black Death. Then, religious mandates stood in the way of opening a dead body to examine its interior. Prohibitions persist today, watered down as social norms.

Right now, the Covid-19 dead must be permitted to speak. Death must reveal, through autopsy, what the last fraught hours of life fought hard to conceal.

As of 29 May 2020, with the official global death toll at 362,238, there were three published reports of autopsies.

The facts in this chapter are from those reports.

When I began reading these reports, I felt the same shiver of fear and expectation I experienced years ago as a resident attending an autopsy of a patient I had cared for. This pandemic has made every event in every victim an intimacy. Each anecdote of suffering is tactile, synaesthetic. Very nearly—experience.

As I read, I am an undergraduate, back in the glass-roofed hall that has sheltered the dead since the 1880s. I hear again the disparaging gurgles of resident pigeons, clustered on the high rafters, jostling for a closer look at the dead. I smell the cold reek of formalin, carbolic and blood. The floor is channelled for drainage. As a slab is hosed down, the marble floor is veined pink. I see all this, knowing the autopsy I'm about to witness took place in very different surroundings in real time.

On the slab before me is Hans, a seventy-five-year-old man. I have his details on the case file, and I will match them against the body's revelations. While I have been reading the narrative of his illness, the man's body has been opened with a standard midline incision, and I get my first view of the focus of disease. The lungs.

They look grey and boggy. Lifted out of the chest cavity, they prove heavy. Together they weigh nearly 3 kg. They would have weighed one-fourth of that when Hans was in good health.

Fluid has displaced all the air within the lungs, giving them a near solid consistency. Sliced through, they will cut as smooth, solid and gelatinous as liver. The old-fashioned label for this change is 'hepatisation'. The lungs have lost their elasticity because the alveolar walls are turgid with inflammation. Hans would have felt a growing difficulty in breathing. The sheer work of moving the chest wall would have exhausted him.

A closer look tells me the surface of Hans's lungs aren't the smooth, regular purplish-grey they seemed at first glance. Bluish areas alternate with crimson patches. I must wait for microscopy to explain this.

The blood vessels of the lungs have a clot. That could have been what finally killed Hans.

There are blood clots in the deep veins of the left leg too. Was this a separate disease, or did COVID-19 cause it?

The rest of Hans looks as normal as a dead man can be expected to look. His organs have been removed now to be sectioned for microscopy. While waiting to peer at them, I review his CT scans. The 'ground glass' appearance of his lung fields is so familiar, it's almost a meme. After having seen his lungs for real, the CT seems a gross understatement.

Under the microscope, the lung shows signs of diffuse alveolar destruction. The alveoli are lined by a hyaline deposit that looks like a membrane. The alveolar cavity is a mess of webbed protein and entrapped cells. The mottled appearance is now explained as islands of cell death caused by microthrombi. The alveolar walls bulge, boggy with inflammation. This lung has no space left for air. What else could Hans have experienced but ARDS?

Hans also had other problems. He is obese. He has had several heart attacks, and his coronary arteries feel plasticised. None of these troubles killed him. But did they push Covid-19 into ARDS?

I'm told viral particles were isolated mainly from the lungs. Other organs had a smattering of virus, and there was a very mild presence of virus in the blood.

That's all I've learned this morning from the Book of the Dead.

I know that other patients have died with troubles very different from Hans. I want to look at their brains, their kidneys, their hearts to understand the travels of SARS-CoV-2. I want to learn how to stop it from destroying the body—piecemeal or in the tsunami of disaster that follows a cytokine storm.

I am not equipped to think up therapies, but I am equipped to think, as are you.

Every death is a tragedy and must be dealt with sensitivity and respect for the wishes of the departed. Surely the dead will want to have suffered to some avail, to relieve, even if only in death, the suffering of others.

The Book of the Dead must be read 'To make his soul flourish, to prevent him from dying a second time'.

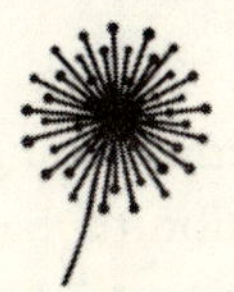

28
The Sanity Clause

The crisis has just passed.
Uh oh, here it comes again,
looking for someone to blame itself on, you, I...
– John Ashbery, *Laughing Gravy*, 1998

Insanity is a deal breaker. Any agreement must carry a sanity clause. If one of the parties is non compos mentis, the deal is void.

We once had a deal with the virus.

The coronavirus was part of the landscape millions of years before we emerged as human. For millennia, we barely noticed each other. When we eventually acknowledged viruses, just a hundred years ago, we got curious about them. We scrutinised the virus and thought our findings true—which they are, but only from our point of view.

Solipsism defines our species. We are self-absorbed to the exclusion of all else. For what could be the purpose of all else but to serve our own? Our anthropocentric universe does not converse. It only demands and commands. If short-changed or crossed, it retaliates with violence.

If our responses as a species were to be embodied in an individual, it won't require a psychiatrist to name the problem. The guy on the street will do that with a loud: 'Mental!'

To me, the most frightening thing about COVID-19 is not ARDS. It is the conjunction of barbarity and credulity that has resulted in a collective suspension of disbelief.

This morning, at 6 a.m., I ventured out to buy milk. I wore a mask—not because it made any scientific sense in an uncontaminated zone but because there was a government order threatening me with arrest if I didn't.

The road was empty. Fruit, vegetable and milk vendors were open for business, but I was the only customer in sight. Everybody was masked. Some masks covered an ear, some the neck, one was pushed back on the forehead. A havaldar, strolling lathi in hand, had pulled his mask aside to bargain over tomatoes. Chai made its rounds. We greedily absorbed this interlude of camaraderie before the havaldar could adjust his mask and swing his lathi. Dour and silent, we relished that brief truce before the virus repossessed our lives.

A woman leaned out of a second-floor balcony and yelled at me: 'Don't walk!'

'Why?' I yelled back.

She slapped her forehead at my ignorance. 'You'll catch the virus!'

'How?'

'It's on the ground, no? Goes right through your shoes. Even Nikes! It's got spikes!'

The dewy morning was fragrant with unseen flowers. Somewhere, a koel sang her heart out. But the set faces around me weren't fooled one bit. All of them had information streaming in live from the—the—you know, right? They knew all about the conspiracy.

The air, the ground, the trees, the birds, the flowers, the passing zephyr, even the lazy sun—all of them were at it already, churning out viruses in free fall.

Spring passed over us, unnoticed.

Where do we even begin? Either admit this is the end of reason or else, see reason. And the only form reason can take now is science. It is our only rescue from paranoia and the violence inherent to it.

That violence is implicit in the language of COVID-19. Take the commonest phrase in use today: 'social distancing'. What does it mean?

Of course, everybody knows what it means: to keep out of the range of droplet infection. In Florida, it means keeping an alligator-length apart.

The correct term would have been 'physical distancing'. Which is the simple, hygienic precaution of physical containment. It is a form of self-awareness that promotes grace of movement, delicacy of touch, sensitivity to the company present. It is inherent to every culture, but really it has nothing to do with culture at all.

It has everything to do with negotiating co-existence.

It is a declaration of intent:

I'm not getting in your way.

I won't touch you unless you want me to.

You don't have to smell the garlic on my breath.

I won't spray you with my saliva.

And all that, in expectation of reciprocity. It is just common decency. But it also enhances communication because of the sensitivity displayed. It is a position of trust.

Social distancing is the exact opposite. It is a position of mistrust. It has everything to do with negotiating alienation. It is what happens when lockdown continues after the virus threat has passed. A forcible subjugation and segregation of human beings.

India has a 3,000-year-old tradition of this. We have a caste system. We love eugenics and practice it in many subtle ways.

Though ascribed to religion, these ideas have no roots in the institution. Religion itself is rooted in human behaviour.

And human behaviour is dictated by the body's urgencies. I'm certain the caste system originated under a disease threat like this one. Physical distancing may have worked—but it very quickly became social distancing, codified as accepted behaviour. What began as simple directive became malevolent and exploitable, creating and defining class. This happened because it was based on exclusion and isolation. The two leading global strategies against Covid-19 are the same, aren't they? The ridiculous ideas of 'purity', common to all world cultures, also have their roots in a dread of contagion.

We can see it in action today. People have been forced out of their homes or barricaded within, beaten up, denied shelter and food and basic necessities. On what suspicion? Of having come from infected countries, of having infected friends, of *maybe*—just maybe, because who's got the test anyway—being Covid-19-positive.

Having lost jobs and shelter, migrant workers have walked hundreds of miles along highways, their meagre possessions bundled, children riding on their shoulders, trudging the miles, certain of refuge when they reach the village they think of as home. Only to be beaten back, refused entry from the dread of contagion.

It takes no time at all to regard your neighbour as dangerous. Othering begins in dread, and finds its expression in violence impossible to imagine till you see it happening.

Paranoia? The term glides glibly off the tongue. It implies a delusional state. But Covid-19 is no delusion. Still, its characterisation is that of the classic imaginary threat. Consider what we believe:

~ It is invisible, ubiquitous and survives on surfaces for hours.

~ It may be shed in all body secretions: tears, saliva, respiratory droplets, urine, stool.

~ It stays for hours on the skin.

~ It can be inhaled, but it also can enter the digestive tract.

Has there ever been a pathogen as all-pervasive, as all-invasive, as mercilessly lethal?

We go out masked and gloved for the briefest possible time, return to a surgical scrub, and in the immortal words of Dylan Thomas, polish the potatoes and, before we let the sun in, mind he wipes his feet.

We do all this in the hope it won't get us, this mysterious spiked ball. That it won't dive into the depths of our lungs, cut off air and choke us to death.

We hope.

There is no cure.

There is no preventive.

Isn't that enough to drive the sanest mind to paranoia?

I think we can and must reason our way out of this. Because, as things stand, no matter which country you live in, the healthcare systems have already buckled under pressure. It is going to take a great deal of individual strength to weather this.

To understand the cause of this pandemic, look again at that crown of thorns.

Yes, it is the coronavirus, but not quite in the way it sounds. Try saying the word with a caesura in the middle—the last syllable a question, as in standard teen-talk—and you'll come closer to the truth.

Like this: coronavirUS?

COVID-19 is not about the virus. It is about the coronavirus and us.

Unfortunately, from the first alarum, the virus has hogged the limelight. Our *STOP THE VIRUS!* strategy isn't working because it ignores the second element in the equation:

Coronavirus + US = COVID-19

The worst news about COVID-19 is its complication: a pneumonia that can kill. ARDS—acute respiratory distress syndrome—is encountered in many other serious illnesses as well. It represents an uncontrolled, and uncontrollable, immune response within the lung.

Why does the body react this way? Numbers and statistics mean nothing. They are constantly in flux.

To make sense of the situation, it is the individual response that is important:

Some people never get sick;
Others do, but very mildly;
Yet others get seriously sick, but recover;
And some die.

The virus infects them all. The outcome depends on how their bodies respond.

This is an epidemic, which is now a pandemic, but we might as well be calling it a plague.

'Epidemic' has resonance; its scientific connotations suggest a backstory of discovery and arouse expectations of prevention and control. It conveys dread, but not helplessness. It implies familiarity and commands action.

In contrast, fatalism is inherent to 'plague'. It suggests a situation that has escalated beyond any possible measure of control. It reinforces panic. It has a secret agenda. It exposes our powerlessness against a larger plan we know nothing about.

Science refutes the word plague in its generic sense. Plague is the disease caused by the bacteria *Yersinia pestis.* And yet, in many ways, we are treating COVID-19 like a plague.

PUBLIC ADVISORY

Every suspected case must be referred to hospital.
Caregivers must be quarantined.
Contacts must be traced.
The house and goods belonging to the infected person must be sealed.
Any caregiver other than those designated ought to be penalised.

Are you wondering why I've included that? Isn't it common cant by now?

True, but I thought the date of that advisory might interest you.

17 January 1348.

That is the first ever public advisory for quarantine. It was issued in Pistoia, Tuscany, in the early weeks of what would soon become the Black Death.

Compare that with the WHO's COVID-19 guidelines, and you'll find very little has changed.

The virus seems to mock us with its ubiquity—how do we stop it?

The information is terrifying.

No longer is the virus restricted to droplets—we read of it being airborne, and that it can be, quite simply, breathed in. We wash our hands in a surgical scrub every half an hour. Our floors are awash with disinfectant. We have been told it sticks to the skin, to every other kind of surface for hours—if so, how do we tell if it is gone?

It is shed in blood and tears and sweat and stools and urine.

All of that could be true.

Equally true: you could breathe in a zillion microbes and stay healthy.

And the reason is—you.

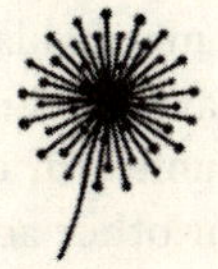

29
Bats and Covid-19

The law of contagion is a magical law that suggests that once two people or objects have been in contact a magical link persists between them unless or until a formal cleansing, consecration, exorcism, or other act of banishing breaks the non-material bond.

– James George Frazer, *The Golden Bough*, 1890

The remarkable fact about the Covid-19 story is how the virus genome was sequenced so very early.

~ On 31 December 2019, Wuhan Municipality reported a cluster of twenty-seven cases of pneumonia.

~ On 7 January 2020, the novel coronavirus, 2019-nCoV (now renamed SARS-CoV-2), was identified as the cause.

~ On 10 January 2020, the genome of this novel virus was made public.

Making the genomic sequence of a virus public is a gift to science—anybody and everybody can then work on the virus. The excellence of a few brains can be extended by a scientific collective of investigation and research.

My admiration for the dedication of Chinese scientists and doctors in their efforts to inform and educate knows no bounds. They have approached, as nearly as is humanly possible, the very quintessence of science.

On sequencing, SARS-CoV-2 was found to approximate the bat coronavirus RaTG13.

Very soon, scientists were investigating the evolution of the genome by applying the molecular clock to track its most recent common ancestor. This helped pinpoint the actual date of the 'emergence' of the novel coronavirus. The result was surprising: there were two, not one, strains of SARS-CoV-2 in circulation.

The virus had emerged 91–214 days before reportage. Within this period, it had diverged from the host (animal) strain and acquired distinctive characters that defined it as a novel coronavirus, capable of infecting humans. The authors of this study raised the possibility that the Wuhan wet market might not have been the only source of spillover.

Much of what the world knows about China's bats and their viruses derives from the work of Dr Shi Zhengli, affectionately called China's 'bat woman'. Dr Shi has explored caves and sampled bats for viruses for years. Here are some observations from her group of researchers:

Following the SARS epidemic of 2002–03, SARSrCoV[13] was isolated first in masked palm civets and raccoon dogs, and subsequently in the Chinese horseshoe bat, *Rhinolophus sinicus*. SARSrCoV uses the same receptor as SARS-CoV for cell entry—ACE2.

Bats sampled from other countries also had SARSrCoV, which also used ACE2.

This fixed the bat as the host reservoir for SARS-CoV. Palm civets and raccoon dogs were intermediate hosts—incidental, perhaps.

It seemed right to conclude that there are SARS-related coronaviruses circulating in bats globally, and some of them use the ACE2 receptor for cell entry.

But can these bat viruses directly affect humans without an intermediary host?

---

13. Severe acute respiratory syndrome-related coronavirus.

Shitou Cave, on the outskirts of Kunming, the capital of Yunnan province, is densely colonised by bats. Dr Shi has sampled bats there since 2011 and isolated SARSrCoVs from them. Yunnan did not have any cases of SARS in the two outbreaks of 2002 and 2004.

In 2015, researchers sampled 208 villagers who lived within the ambit of the bats of Shitou Cave and who also regularly handled wild livestock. Six of these people had antibodies to SARSrCoV. None of them had any respiratory complaints. The antibodies proved that they had, in the past, been affected by SARSrCoV. *So, a spillover had occurred directly from bats into a surrounding human population.*

To me, this is illustrative of how insidiously, and unobtrusively, spillovers can occur. Not all of them cause outbreaks of zoönoses, even if they do cause infections. The same phenomenon was observed by the earliest workers in Uganda's Zika Forest in the 1950s.

Although SARSrCoV is seen as the precursor to SARS-CoV, there are too many genetic differences between them to look at them with linearity. It was only in 2013 that a bat SARSrCoV that uses the ACE2 receptor was isolated. This provided the strongest evidence of the bat origin of SARS-CoV.

Dr Shi's group's five-year surveillance of bats in the Shitou Cave found a wide variation in the SARSrCoVs. There was a close resemblance between some of the variants and human SARS-CoV.

This suggested that the SARS outbreak that emerged in Guangdong may have originated in Yunnan. Genetically, it seemed likely that the evolution of the virus was closely linked to geographic location. The cave was a typical bat hangout—many types of bats congregated there in the mating season. Recombination events would have been fast and furious—and, hey presto—spillover!

It is worthwhile here to pause and consider the different kinds of coronaviruses circulating in bats. Of the four genera of coronaviruses, alpha and beta coronaviruses infect only mammals; gamma and delta coronaviruses infect mostly birds. The target tissue of alpha and beta coronaviruses is respiratory in us humans, but usually intestinal in other mammals. Of the coronaviruses found in humans, there are three we know can be lethal: SARS-CoV, MERS-CoV and, now, SARS-CoV-2. The other human CoVs (HCoV-NL63, HCoV-229E, HCoV-OC43 and HKU1) *mostly* cause mild infections. The qualifier is necessary: we don't, yet, know if they can mutate into more virulent forms.

Bats are the most likely natural reservoirs of alpha and beta coronaviruses. This is very far from being a purely Chinese observation: *Rhinolophus* bats from Europe and other parts of Asia also have variants of SARS-CoV.

The association between bats and coronaviruses is evolutionary and ancient. The fact that it has been so carefully conserved indicates a high degree of mutual benefit.

Judging from the enormous number of variants of SARSrCoVs found in bats in Shitou Cave, it has been concluded that SARS-CoV arose from a recombination event between SARSrCoV, the principal bat coronavirus, and another unidentified virus. If so, this scenario may be commoner than we think. Bat congregations are everywhere—I can name five such sites offhand within a 5 km radius of my home, and I live in the frenetically paced heart of India's largest city.

It is interesting that, during the SARS outbreak of 2002–03, there were no cases in Yunnan, near the cave where the virus presumably originated. How can that be explained?

Enter the intermediate host. In this case, the masked palm civet cat, an animal that was popular merchandise at that Guangdong market, the evident favourite with the province's most innovative chefs. The masked palm civet, *Paguma larvata,* is a native of the Himalayas and Southeast Asia. It acted as an amplifying host for the newly emerged SARS-CoV.

How did *Paguma* acquire the virus? Very likely on a farm frequented by bats, or a farm which had displaced a bat habitat. Or, it could have acquired it from another, earlier, intermediate host, as yet unnamed. It is likely that, after it made the species jump, SARS-CoV underwent changes that increased its virulence. The newly changed genes may have coded for proteins that can block vital steps in innate immunity.

Besides the human infections of SARS, MERS and Covid-19, another zoönosis has recently emerged from bat coronaviruses—this affects pigs, causing swine acute diarrhoea syndrome.

The refrain of bat coronaviruses-related zoönoses, all emerging in China, led a group of researchers to state in a paper published in March 2019:

> Thus, it is highly likely that future SARS- or MERS-like coronavirus outbreaks will originate from bats, and there is an increased probability that this will occur in China. Therefore, the investigation of bat coronaviruses becomes an urgent issue for the detection of early warning signs, which in turn minimizes the impact of such future outbreaks in China.

Bat coronaviruses seem to cluster by genera. SARSrCoV is present in many species of bats, but all of them belong to two families—Rhinolophidae and Hipposideradae.

Old World bats[14] are not represented in the Americas. But in 2007, researchers in Colorado examined fifty-seven bats from the Rocky Mountain region and discovered copious coronavirus RNA in their faecal deposits too. These were apparently healthy bats, but the fact that their faecal shedding of virus was so high suggests they are probably reservoir hosts, just like their eastern cousins.

Many of the North American bats that harbour coronaviruses are, like their Chinese counterparts, urbanised. They roost in buildings and barns, and they too interface with humans. But compared to eastern bats, we don't know much about the coronaviruses circulating in them. Bats from Mexico also contain a rich treasury of coronaviruses.

There are 1,200 species of bats. There are as many or perhaps more coronaviruses.

How are we going to keep track of them all?

Bat surveillance is arduous and dangerous. I think it might also be self-defeating. Nothing in nature is quite as linear as human logic.

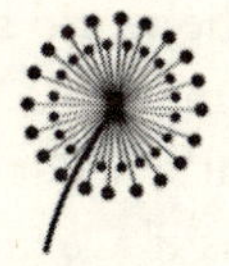

14. Members of the family *Pteropodidae* are known colloquially as flying foxes, mega-bats or Old World fruit bats. The family is composed of 41 genera and about 170 species.

30

Spillover!

Cry 'Havoc!,' and let slip the dogs of war.

– William Shakespeare, *Julius Caesar*

As a single word, used to describe just what it sounds like, an overflow, 'spillover' was first used in the 1940s. It was convenient coinage—in economics, in politics—an excuse for military mishaps which could *spillover* into civilian damage.

One of the first things a surgical resident learns is to shun the word 'inadvertent'. Accidents, we're taught, are simply awareness failures. In its early career, 'spillover' seemed reserved for such situations. It was irresponsibility brought to the table, elegant in aspic, when facts grew too hard to digest.

It was a word I loathed even more when it grew vertebrate and took on the world as a zoönosis.

'Zoönosis' irritated me too. 'Zoögnosis' would have been more apt, for what's needed now and forever, is a gnosis of other life forms if we are to save our own.

In this time of Covid-19, spillover and zoönosis are practically conjoined twins. The two words are yoked together by a third: emergence.

1. The pathogen circulates in a reservoir host.

2. A spillover occurs, leading to the infection of either an intermediate host or vector, or the direct infection of humans.

3. A pathogen that has not been encountered before 'emerges' and is termed novel. SARS-CoV-2 is a 'novel

virus' that has emerged as a zoönosis by a spillover from bats.

What does spillover mean? How does it occur? Why should it occur at all when the virus has an easy ride in the reservoir host? These questions are vital to this pandemic—and to the next.

We know, hitherto, that the bat is the reservoir host for SARS-CoV-2, just as it was for SARS-CoV-1 and MERS-CoV. With this background, here are the dynamics of the virus's spillover.

On the one hand is the bat, with a stable population of circulating viruses.

On the other, is a healthy human population.

For years, perhaps centuries, they've coexisted without disease. Suddenly then, without warning, without notice, there is a spillover.

'Without notice' simply means 'we have yet to notice'.

Look at what we have noticed already. For decades, scientists have been studying zoönoses of various kinds. These observations identify three phases:

Phase 1: Pathogen pressure. The amount of pathogen circulating in the host, the time and place and method of pathogen release, the survival of the shed virus outside the host, the agencies of spread and its range of action.

Phase 2: The human–host interface. This depends on host and human behaviour, and how they engage with each other. This is what determines the human exposure to the pathogen.

Phase 3: The disease outcome. What is the course of the zoönosis? Is it a mild infection? Is it a killer? This depends on the human host's reaction to the invading pathogen. This, in turn, depends on the genetic and immunological status of the patient and the dose and route of exposure to the pathogen.

The story of Covid-19, too, will be scripted along these lines, from bat to pandemic.

Pandemics do not happen—until they do. So, what prevents pandemics from happening?

A mismatch at every step keeps reservoir host and human barricaded from each other and well apart—until they fall in step. Such alterations in rhythm can scarcely follow linear logic. Unpredictable as this sounds, there are mathematical models for spillover built around this.

The first factor is the viral population in the reservoir host. When does it increase? What determines this increase? What controls the amount of virus shed?

Bats aggregate in the thousands for birthing. As a pattern of social behaviour, they roost in a huddle through rough times or through winters. At such times, different species of bats intermingle. They carry different viruses, of course, and these social gatherings offer an opportunity for viruses to change through recombination. Replication is also stepped up in such congenial conditions. Large RNA viruses lack a 'proofreading' mechanism, so as replication increases, so do 'errors', and 'unedited' genomes abound in mutations, which may change the virulence of the virus. Thus, at any time, not only can the circulating population of viruses change in density, it can also change in character.

After replication, the virus's agenda is dispersal. How far can it go, and how many fresh hosts can it infect? This depends on how it is shed from the reservoir host, and how it survives in the environment.

Rabies virus is shed in the saliva. In carnivores, biting behaviour assures virus dispersal, so successful dispersal demands a concentration of the virus in the salivary gland.

Dengue and Zika viruses, after maturing in the digestive system of the mosquito, are concentrated in the salivary glands and directly injected into the skin when the mosquito bites us.

Coronaviruses are shed in bat excrement.

Once it has left the body of the reservoir host, the pathogen pressure a virus can build up or dissipate for infectivity depends largely on the environment in which it finds itself. If it is shed directly into the environment, how long can it survive on various surfaces? How long can it survive on fomites?[15] Can it survive in water? Can it be blown about by the wind?

In addition, environmental factors might completely disconnect the virus from the host—so the actual area of virus dispersal, and therefore of infectivity, may be well beyond the host's ambit. We see an example of this every monsoon in Bombay, when the roads are flooded with water from choked drains and gutters and there are outbreaks of leptospirosis. *Leptospira*, the pathogen responsible, is shed in the urine of rodents. Transported by the flooding, *Leptospira* travels way beyond the ambit of the rat whose original libation it was.

Viral shedding and human behaviour present an important conjunct to pathogen pressure by magnifying contact. Animal and bird slaughter often approximates a massacre, with indiscriminate spillage and handling of the viscera. Under such conditions, the human–host interface is intensified. If this coincides with a period of increased viral shedding by the host, the pathogen pressure can exceed limits and cause a spillover.

---

15. From the Latin '*fomes*', meaning tinder. It refers to materials or objects likely to carry infection—such as clothes, utensils, furniture.

Consider the invasion of a bat roost by urban development. Thousands of bats are displaced, perhaps at a point in time when they are particularly pathogen-enriched. The spread of viral shedding is unimaginable as they hastily regroup. Many of their new roosts will be urban, within residential areas, gardens or large public spaces.

Bats are a common feature in most roofed public spaces like railway stations. Their hangouts are human hangouts too. While this may be ignored as a part of the usual landscape most of the time, it becomes ominous when host conditions are conducive for spillover. High-intensity exposures, however brief, are more likely to cause spillover than low-dose exposures over extended periods.

The next phase is the actual process of infection. When one considers the ubiquity of pathogens, we humans seem to do a smart job of evading infections. We dabble daily in horrendous pathogens—viruses, bacteria, protozoa, fungi, prions, particulate toxins, things we don't even know by name. Yet, they leave us unscathed. When there is a spillover, this complacence is deeply shaken.

The human body has as many defences as a virus has tricks. It is this cat-and-mouse game that decides the establishment of a zoönosis. Can its outcome be predicted?

This depends as much on individual human factors as on the exposure to the virus.

I think a relevant question might be: can we identify the population at risk?

At first, this seems self-evident. The most susceptible are people who are at the forefront of the virus–human interface: butchers, leather workers, farmers, poachers, toddy tappers—the list is endless. Yes, these people are obviously vulnerable, but how do you explain infections in people unconnected with such exposure?

People in the first group are exposed to high doses of the pathogen. People in the second group are infected even without that intense exposure. What's the difference? Has the virulence of the pathogen increased by the time it reaches the second group? Or does something in that second group make them more vulnerable to infection?

Both may be equally true.

Most pathogens, once they have spilt over, rapidly increase in virulence. If the host–human jump establishes human-to-human transmission, the virus often changes in virulence and infectivity. Human-to-human transmission also depends on the route of viral shedding, and the survival of the virus between human hosts. Respiratory viruses like coronaviruses, spread by droplet infection, can be inhaled, and this widens the ring of contagion.

But the second possibility is something I think should be considered, especially in a pandemic of this sort, where everyone everywhere seems to be infected. Are we at increased risk because something has changed in *us*? Has something made our innate immunity shaky, making us more vulnerable to a respiratory infection?

COVID-19 can turn downright dangerous: yesterday's mild cough is today's wheeze is tomorrow's desperate struggle to breathe as pneumonia sets in. And no ordinary pneumonia this. This can end in the worst respiratory emergency known to us: ARDS. It is a bad situation—and what do you think causes it? The virus?

Nah.

Sure, the virus started the illness. But this, this nasty complication that can kill, is a reaction of the patient's own body. It is a response of uncontrolled, and uncontrollable, immunity.

There you have it. The cause of death in Covid-19 is… suicide.

So what brings this about?

ARDS is not unique to Covid-19. It is the end-stage complication in a wide variety of insults to the body:

~ Trauma.

~ Direct chemical injury to the lung, through inhaled toxins or aspirated stomach contents high in acid.

~ Infections.

How do we stop this complication of uncontrolled immunity, which results in uncontrollable inflammation?

The desperate effort to save patients with Covid-19, which occupies every doctor's thoughts today, is centred on that question.

No, I have no answer, but I do have a thought I'd like you to consider, in the hope that *you* might be the one to find the answer to that question.

But before we exchange that thought, we must look closer at how the coronavirus may have spilt over from bats.

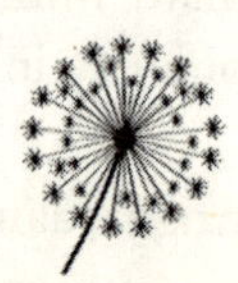

31

The Reservoir Host

The books stood open and the gates unbarred...
The future was a verb in hibernation.

– Seamus Heaney, *Villanelle for an Anniversary*, 1986

The horseshoe bat (*Rhinolophus sinicus*) has been identified as the reservoir host for SARS-CoV-2. It is also the reservoir host for SARS-CoV and MERS-CoV—and for a number of other coronaviruses.

Bats were among the earliest mammals to evolve, at the beginning of the Eocene, some 50 million years ago. That was a period when global temperatures shot up to equal, if not exceed, the global temperatures today. We are, presently, on a 50 million year retro trip in climate change, one likely to peak at its warmest ever by 2030.

I think it is an important parallel to notice during a pandemic. It may have given the bat a distinctive relationship with an equally ancient organism: the virus.

Bats haven't changed much over the last 50 million years. Nor, perhaps, has their association with viruses. Bats and the viruses they carry may have co-evolved. This suggests that viruses use receptors and biochemical pathways which have been conserved in more recently evolved mammals. It is an important clue in understanding the susceptibility of various host species today.

How many viruses do bats carry?

We have no idea. So far, sixty-six disease-causing, bat-borne viruses are known. There could be a hundred more.

Bats (Chiroptera) are everywhere. They have two large suborders, appropriately dubbed 'Yin' and 'Yang'. Yinpterochiroptera includes both bats that echolocate and those that don't. All Yangopterochiroptera bats echolocate. Echolocation is the unique ability to navigate through the use of sound. Bat sounds are mostly ultrasonic—beyond the range of the human ear. But some of them can be loud enough to deafen us. These sounds, produced by the larynx under considerable abdominal muscular effort, spray forth aerosols of virus-rich saliva.

Yinpterochiroptera and Yangopterochiroptera parted company soon after they evolved. Except for the poles, there is no part of the planet where bats don't abound. As the only extant flying mammal, the bat is something of an evolutionary wonder.

Bats of *Myotis* species may travel 200 to 400 miles from their winter hibernation sites. Brazilian and Mexican free-tailed bats (*Tadarida brasiliensis mexicana*) are the most abundant mammals in the Americas. They summer in New Mexico and Texas, then winter in Mexico—an 800 mile flight between vacation spots. These are just two examples of the vagility of bats, but they convey an idea of how far bat-borne viruses can travel.

A bat is a contradiction in terms: a furred, leather-winged bird; a vampire that suckles its young. This fruitarian gourmand is large-hearted too: neighbours are welcome to share leftovers. Species no bar—as long as they don't object to a rich jus of bat saliva.

Bats nap their way through periods of stress by the inbuilt response of sopor and torpor, when they switch to a lower metabolic rate to conserve energy.

Bats have long lifespans and low birth rates. In this they break an evolutionary rule: usually, the smaller the animal, the briefer its life span and the higher its brith rate.

Bats delight in oral sex. The short-nosed fruit bats (*Cynopterus sphinx*) fancy fellatio, while the Indian flying foxes (*Pteropus medius*) incline to cunnilingus.

Don't believe me? Unfortunately, the videos on National Geographic are no longer watchable. As necessary moral policing in this time of Covid-19, they have been removed for violating YouTube's policy on nudity and sexual content.

For all the noise about bats, we know very little about them—and next to nothing when it comes to the deal between bats and coronaviruses. The one thing we do know is that, despite their heavy viral load, bats don't fall sick very often.

In many ways, a bat is virus heaven:

Sociable: Bats congregate in the thousands, offering plenty of opportunities for interaction with other viruses and thus for recombination.

Vagile: Bats fly shorter distances than birds, true, but flight is a great route for viral dispersal—not just across a city but across geographical borders as well.

Long-lived: Not a host that will turn a virus out into the cold without notice, this one! The virus can set up its replication machinery and keep xeroxing itself with nary a thought for the morrow.

Species no bar: Jam-packed with busily circulating viruses, bats can disperse them across a wide range of hosts. Spillovers, here they come!

Immunity: Bats have evolved, along with flight, a high tolerance to many widely divergent viruses. Welcome aboard!

Sopor and torpor: Many bats are able to do this for long periods of time under stress conditions. Think of it as a bat lockdown—the viruses hunker down and wait it out.

So when the bat wakes up to normalcy, viral shedding is back with a zing, increasing the possibility of prolonged or repeated infectivity.

Fever and flight: Bats jumpstart the energy demands of flight by raising body temperature. This means their viral passengers have evolved strategies to stay alive at higher temperatures. In most organisms, fever is an important defence against infection; it starts off the immune process. Viruses that deplane after a hot flight on a bat may not be impressed by the immune response of their next host.

Here's the manifest of scary bat-borne viruses:

~ *Lyssaviruses*, of which rabies virus is the most frightening human threat, also have their natural home in bats. All Lyssaviruses attack nervous tissue across a wide variety of hosts. Transmission is through the saliva. Most mammals succumb to rabies, except for the reservoir host. Bats have circulating antibody against rabies virus.

~ *Paramyxoviruses*, of which we've known two in recent times:

1. Hendra virus was limited to Australia, where it emerged in horses infected by bat urine. The humans affected were ostlers, horse handlers. Till today, there have been five spillover events, with seven human deaths.

2. Nipah virus, the recent killer virus on the Indian subcontinent and in Southeast Asia. It emerged in Malaysia in 1999, among pig handlers. Guano from bats roosting in barns first infected pigs. Pig handlers developed fever that quickly turned into fatal encephalitis and coma. Nipah virus emergence in Bangladesh is very well documented. Bats and humans share a love for date-palm toddy. In most villages, the pot left on the tree to collect the drip of the delicious sap was also a nocturnal pit stop for bats. When humans

imbibed their share, it was a rich soup of bat saliva, full of Nipah virus. Once it emerged as a human infection, human-to-human transmission was rapid. The disease carries an alarmingly high fatality rate.

~ *Coronaviruses*, of which bats have 200 types (at the last count). Of the bat virome that has been sequenced, coronaviruses make up 35 per cent.

SARS emerged in 2002 in a market in Guangdong province, China. It was soon traced to a common merchandise—palm civets—sold in Chinese markets as a delicacy. Raccoon dogs, also on sale, had the virus too. These incidental or accidental hosts led the SARS-CoV trail back to bats.

As predicted, once the species jump occurred, human-to-human transmission was very rapid. Bats of many species have antibodies to this highly pathogenic virus. This may be of great relevance in our present epidemic.

In 2012, MERS emerged in the Middle East as a pneumonia with a very high complication and mortality rate. The Egyptian tomb bat (*Taphozous perforatus*) carried a virus that corresponded with the human virus isolate completely. It is now believed that the intermediate host in this epidemic was the camel. Antibodies to MERS-CoV are found in camels of the Arabian Peninsula and North Africa. Most human cases can be traced back to contact with camels or camel products. Studies suggest that camels have been circulating MERS-CoV at least since the 1980s.

MERS-CoV has not been isolated from bats easily. Direct transmission from bats-to-humans is therefore unlikely.

~ *Filoviruses,* which cause fatal hemorrhagic fevers, also circulate in bats.

1. In 2007, Marburg virus emerged in a cave in Uganda that had been colonised by Egyptian fruit bats (*Rousettus*

aegypticus). Miners working in the vicinity developed a haemorrhagic fever, and Marburg virus was directly isolated from these bats.

2. Ebola emerged in 2004 from animals slaughtered for bush meat: gorillas, chimpanzees and duikers—a sub-Saharan antelope. Since then, human-to-human transmission has become more rapid and lethal. Antibodies to Ebola virus have been isolated in a number of bat species, but not the virus. The bat's role as Ebola's reservoir remains speculative.

Very little is known about the bat's tolerance for its teeming viruses.

Bats are hunted madly in many countries. Additionally, in a mistaken attempt to 'eradicate' rabies, large killing pogroms have been carried out in foolhardy attempts to eradicate this natural reservoir host.

The result? Swifter re-emergence, perhaps of a species with increased pathogenicity.

Contrast this with the intelligent and dedicated effort to contain Nipah virus in Bangladesh. Door-to-door education across villages has marshalled a nation of conservationists.

A taste for bat meat too continues to power the vendetta against bats. Culling bats merely shifts the viral population to a new host. Worse, it encourages the emergence of new, lethal strains.

More insidiously, it is the encroachment of bat habitats that spells the emergence of new diseases. In Central and South America, habitat destruction has led to a change of diet in vampire bats. Earlier, these bats fed on sylvan animals. Now, they attack livestock and domestic animals. Similarly, flower and fruit bats transfer their allegiance to agricultural land when forests are cut down for farming.

Spillover events occur when the levels of circulating virus exceed the 'normal' for the reservoir host. The population dynamics of the reservoir host should be the basis of predicting spillovers. This is likely to depend on more than the species of bat. Changing climate, topography and human encroachment on habitats: these lead to changes in the seasonal rhythms of bats.

Growing urbanisation has turned the bat into a metropolitan. Large, busy cities sequester bat populations in residential areas—not just in trees, but inside buildings and in large public spaces that offer roost and viand. Like us, the bat too makes choices of convenience and comfort.

If it helps to change our attitude towards this marvellous mammal, I offer the usual lame plea: *we need bats.*

We need them to pollinate and re-seed land we have deforested.

We need their technology to further our own.

We need their guano to invent new organic fuels and fertilisers.

Above all, we need their magnificence and their beauty to inspire us to look at their world of viruses with less dread and more intelligence.

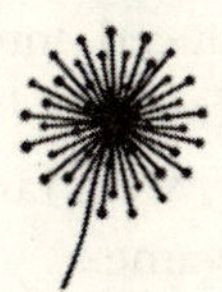

32

The Intermediate Host

Petit à petit, l'oisseau fait son nid.

– French adage

The raccoon dog, *Nyctereutes procyonoides*,[16] is a canid—a dog, not a raccoon. The 'raccoon' label derives from its stripy fur. In Japan, it has a neat niche in folklore as *tanuki*, the shapeshifter. It is a strange canid in many ways. It climbs trees. It feeds on berries. It hibernates. Most importantly, in this time of Covid-19, it has a near-insatiable wanderlust. Its locomotion, in zoological terms, is described as 'cursorial', which suggests a speedy runner, but in the last century the raccoon dog has moved in a leisurely amble across continents.

The Chinese raccoon dog has a transcontinental ambit. Its northern range extends to southeast Siberia, to the valleys of the Amur and Ussuri rivers, where a subspecies, the Ussuri raccoon dog, flourishes. In the 1920s, 9,100 Ussuri dogs were introduced into western Russia. Their acclimatisation to the extreme cold made them luxuriously furry and fat. Initially they were farmed, but they were soon released into the wild as game.

Despite challenges to survival, by the 1950s, Ussuri dogs had sauntered across geographical barriers, climate zones and nations. In 2009, 176,000 raccoon dogs were hunted in Finland. In 2009, Germany's 'hunting bag' figure was

---

16. From the Greek *nukt-*, night + *ereutēs*, wanderer + *prokuōn*, 'before-dog' + *-oidēs*, similar to. The name comes from its superficial resemblance to the raccoon (*Procyon lotor*), to which it is not related.

listed at 30,000. Like Hannibal, and without thirty-eight elephants, raccoon dogs have crossed the Alps and made their way into Italy. They have ambled through Greece and Macedonia. And all that's in the wild. The raccoon dog's fate in human domesticity and care is bloodier by far.

In 2014, the global fur industry was a $40 billion enterprise. China traded 14 million raccoon dog pelts that year alone. In the years that have followed, the world's appetite for fur has fallen—except in China. China is still the world's biggest producer, exporter, importer and consumer of furs—and a large proportion of these are raccoon dog pelts.

Russia was at the forefront of the fur trade for years. 'Murmansky fur trim' is still advertised widely on fashion websites. 'Faux fur' was exposed as raccoon dog pelts not long ago, but the trade continues to flourish.

The raccoon dog is an intermediate host for coronaviruses, and was clearly implicated in the SARS outbreak of 2003. This means it engages with coronaviruses that link up with ACE2 receptors, so it is an animal to be surveilled. Its vagility across Europe, its ease in both sylvan and suburban habitats and its hibernation through extreme cold, make it an ambulant incubator for spillovers.

Hubei province is the principal site for raccoon dog farming. It produces more than 60 per cent of the annual output of pelts. Covert alliances with Western fashion houses and the ever-present consumer keep this demand high. Wuhan, in particular, is a burgeoning market for furs.

Despite legislation and ethical norms, the condition of animals on farms is unspeakable. Chemical assaults to promote fur growth, overcrowded cages and dangerous feeds compound the misery of creatures bred for the express purpose of being killed. Nor is death anodyne. A brief quote here will suffice:

> Skinning begins with a knife at the rear of the belly whilst the animal is lying on its back or hung upside-down by its hind legs from a hook. A significant number of animals remain fully conscious during this process. Helpless, they struggle and try to defend themselves to the very end. Even after their skin has been stripped off, breathing, heart beat, directional body and eyelid movements were evident for 5 to 10 minutes.[17]

The 'humane' solution to 'skinning alive' is to first stun the animal by dashing its head against a brick wall before reaching for the flaying knife.

I should state here, with emphasis, that *these are not practices peculiar to China*. They are peculiar to the meat and animal product trade everywhere in the world.

The exposure of workers in this industry to coronaviruses, which are shed during the flaying and slaughter, must be the most intense known.

A thought for the pangolin, now.

Pangolins are among the most prized mammals in the illegal animal trade. They are poached both for their meat, which is considered a delicacy, and for their scutes, the specialised scales, which are used in Chinese and African traditional medicine.

On 24 March 2019, the Guangdong Wildlife Rescue Centre received twenty-one live Malayan pangolins from the Anti-smuggling Customs Bureau. Besides the fright and misery of incarceration, most of these animals were

17. 'Merciless Slaughter: the unspeakable horror of China's fur farms', Heinz Lienhard, President, Swiss Animal Protection (SAP); Opening speech, SAP press launch, 1 February 2005, Zurich, Switzerland.

sick with skin lesions. Despite medical care, sixteen died. At post-mortem, their lungs were found inflamed and full of a frothy liquid. Some had enlarged livers and spleens. When the viral diversity of this sick population was studied, the two commonest viruses found were Sendai virus and coronaviruses, of all four groups.

Yes, pangolins circulate coronaviruses.

Is the pangolin an intermediate host for COVID-19?

In October 2019, pangolin-CoV—the coronavirus isolated from the lungs of pangolins—was found to be 91.02 per cent identical with SARS-CoV-2, and 90.5 per cent identical with the bat coronavirus RaTG13. The now infamous S1 protein, which achieves infection through cell entry, is practically the same in pangolin-CoV and in human SARS-CoV-2. Though the furin cleavage site that characterises human SARS-CoV-2 spike protein has not been detected in pangolin-CoV, it is still possible that pangolin-CoV may have the potential for human spillover. All these factors indicate that there is a possibility that the pangolin may be the intermediate host responsible for our present pandemic.

The pangolin's fraught career in the wild may endanger more species than its own. There are four species of pangolin extant (two African and two Asian). Pangolins are hunted and poached and trapped and transported alive. Their eventual destination is usually China, but the transport network runs through Europe and, very often, the Americas.

A trapped animal facing deprivation and cruelty, and growing assured each moment of imminent death, is likely to be offloading viruses briskly. That makes the pangolin's complicated journey from jungle to medicine jar an extended viral spillover.

The pangolin and the raccoon dog are only two known examples of how brutish human interference has increased the potential for viral emergence, for spillover and spread. The detection of coronaviruses in these animals merely tells us they are susceptible to being infected by the reservoir host, the bat.

How many other intermediate hosts are there? How are we going to find them all? Track them all? Surveil them all?

That is just one more paranoid scenario.

Coronaviruses may circulate in any number of species, inoffensive and unnoticed. Most of the time, it requires human agency to effect a spillover.

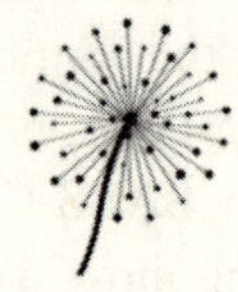

33
A Counter-view

Weep not that the world changes—did it keep
A stable, changeless state, 'twere cause indeed to weep.
– William Cullen Bryant, *Mutation: A Sonnet*, 1824

A square peg in a round hole?

Perhaps it isn't the peg that's awry.

Observations that do not fit the grid aren't necessarily misfits. Nor should they be ignored.

What if we ignore the grid instead?

Lift off the grid through which we view COVID-19, and the vista is different. We must not leave this unexplored.

The Thwack moment—the final day of 2019—defined COVID-19 for us. We saw the disease for the killer it was, exactly as it was described from Wuhan.

On 5 January 2020, the WHO Disease Outbreak News bulletin referred to it as 'Pneumonia of unknown cause—China'. Forty-four people were affected, eleven severely ill. The report went on to add: *The reported link to a wholesale fish and live-animal market could indicate an exposure link to animals.*

That brought 'wet market' into shuddering focus, and it hasn't left the public eye since.

What this pansophical eye hasn't noticed is that *all* markets are wet markets.

Once these lockdowns are lifted, markets will be back with flourish, and I doubt we'll notice that our favourite shopping hot spots are…er…wet.

Our markets sell fish, caught in the wee hours; meat, slaughtered but an hour before; chickens, scuffling to escape the quick cervical dislocation and suffocation in a shopping bag; fruit, vegetables; cookware, spices, flowers. You'll find these cheek by jowl with clothing, trinkets, garden gear and hardware, baking in the noonday sun on a pavement in a Shaniwar Bazaar that's been in action since 1,200 CE, just a stone's throw away from my home. Most pavement markets in small towns and villages are like this one. The covered markets are the same, but they smell worse. Bombay's Crawford Market today has the same pong as Calcutta's New Market did fifty years ago. As a ten-year-old browsing the bookshop, my introduction to Edgar Allan Poe came with a very real whiff of decay. The only difference between these wet markets and your fancy supermarket is tinfoil, plastic, preservatives and iffy climate control. The smell of quiet death leaks past these containment zones.

Wet markets are the way of two-thirds of the planet. Eating a hormone-fed quadruped, stuffed with antibiotics, is not necessarily superior to eating a pig or a jungli weasel. Eat meat, must slaughter.

Vegetarian? Every grain of rice or wheat grows at the cost of a patch of forest—and if you calculate the numbers killed in the process, why, it is mass murder.

So let's drop this manufactured panic about wet markets.

The first patient in Wuhan, a man symptomatic since the first week of December, had no contact with the market in question. Nor had he any contact with an infected person. That suggests SARS-CoV-2 was already around, strolling through Wuhan harmlessly, but with an appointment in Samara.

What made it suddenly dangerous?

What made Covid-19 emerge in Wuhan?

I will examine three factors.

Factor I

Wuhan is a boom town. The building frenzy has altered the cityscape unrecognisably over the last decade. The windswept geography makes it a dustbowl, accumulating deposits from a vast surround.

The result is predictable. The degree of air pollution in the city has long been a concern, and PM2.5 levels have increased since 2014. Much of this fine dust comes from the artificial stone industry and construction sites, and it has a very high silica content. The haze that wrapped Wuhan in December 2019 came mostly from these particulates and vehicular emissions. I think this is of utmost relevance to the emergence of Covid-19.

I consider the troposphere a body part. It is certainly more intimate than any clothing, as it glides in and out of the furthest crevices of my lungs. The term 'ambient air' is used to describe the atmosphere in its natural state, i.e., without pollutants. An irritating term, and semantically wrong. All air is ambient. Unless we exist in a vacuum, air surrounds us on every side. And what is the natural state of air? Who has ever breathed it free of pollutants? Air has been polluted since the planet cooled. Dust is the nature of the beast. So I'll dispense with the qualifier of 'ambient' and get intimate with air.

Originally, 78.09 per cent nitrogen, 20.95 per cent oxygen, 0.93 per cent argon, 0.04 per cent carbon dioxide, plus water vapour. That's what air is meant to be.

None of this is irritant or alien to the lungs. But add to it carbon monoxide, sulphur, lead, nitrous oxide, particulate matter, assorted metals, ozone. Now it is a closer approximate to the true composition of the air we breathe. Deconstructed, a chemistry textbook entire.

Urbanisation has meant the loss of tree cover and the formation of heat islands, where the combustion of petrol and diesel spews organic volatiles and nitrogen dioxide into the air. Ozone is now a common urban pollutant. It is the principal component of smog, which is formed when water vapour, nitrogen dioxide and volatile organic compounds react with each other in strong sunlight.

Pollutants that are water soluble are easily pushed out of the upper airways, and may never make it down to the lungs. Not so ozone. Ozone is a very strong airway irritant. It zooms right in and dissolves in the fluid lining the bronchioles and alveoli, where it reacts with the molecules and cues immune cells into inflammatory responses. While this is happening, we're already coughing and experiencing chest discomfort in the form of a 'tightness'.

Ozone causes long-standing airway inflammation, enough to cripple the normal rhythm of breathing and injure alveolar cells. A mere heartbeat away loom pneumonia, lung disease and respiratory distress. Ozone production, however, needs bright sunlight, so it is highest in the summer months and couldn't have caused much injury in December 2019 in Wuhan.

Instead, the pollutant I worry about most is particulate matter, which is more than just suspended dust. Each particle is a composite, rightly defined as 'a mixture of mixtures'. A particle could be made of all sorts of stuff—from microbes and pollen, to metals and organic molecules and acids, and, of course, the ever-present silica, of various grades. At particle size below 2.5 μm, pollutants reach the alveoli. Smaller particles, termed ultrafine particles, sized below 1 μm, can cross the alveolar/capillary barrier and enter the bloodstream.

Domestic PM2.5 particulates vary with the use of fuel, ventilation, crowding and household activities. Trades like welding, jewellery-making and iron-mongering involve the use of fuels and high temperatures. Others, like milling grain or spices, produce fine dust. Our lungs are the libraries of a lifetime, autobiographies unread.

China is one of the most polluted countries (though, unlike many other nations, it addresses this with some concern). Between 2014 and 2015, a national survey conducted in 190 Chinese cities arrived at these figures for premature deaths attributable to inhaled particulates:

PM2.5 = 722,370

PM10 = 1,491,774

Particulates create micro-weather conditions and concentrate their impact on population clusters, each of which may be exposed to a particular component in greater concentration. Even within a 10 km radius, we do not breath the same air.

The respiratory tree is impacted at every stage of breathing. Many intracellular pathways of inflammation are open to manipulation by particulates. Muco-ciliary clearance gets rid of larger particulates from the lower airways, but the upper airways bear the brunt. While operatic illnesses like nasopharyngeal cancers are quickly acknowledged, humbler ailments like chronic sinusitis, colds and sore throats may be of even greater significance.

The implication of this in SARS-CoV-2 infection is evident.

The upper airway is the site of maximum viral engagement because of its great number of ACE2 receptors. Chronic inflammation here will encourage a pro-inflammatory response to the virus, increasing the likelihood of severe disease.

Smaller PM2.5 particles in the lower airway induce a strongly pro-inflammatory milieu. There is increased production of cytokines, and increased cell death from autophagy and oxidative stress. In addition, as a result of chronic irritation, there may be structural injury to alveolar and capillary cells.

A lung chronically inflamed by particulates, and now infected by a virus, can be rushed into ARDS.

In my view particulates may well have been a deciding factor in the emergence of Covid-19.

Wuhan had a very dismal AQI at the time of this outbreak. It was also bitterly cold in Wuhan.

My long love affair with Jane Austen has forever been tormented by the earliest mention of her death I read. It appeared in the introduction to *Pride and Prejudice*:

Consequent to catching cold, Austen died in Winchester on 18 July 1817 at the age of forty.

At twelve, it devastated me. How could one die of a cold? The question wore me out in torrid Bombay as I sneezed all summer, dripped a rich and bubbling cold when it rained, nurtured a frog in my throat come winter, and still managed to stay very far from death. Finally, I put it down to the dark ages. 1817 was antiquity.

Killing Jane is a popular past time in British medical journals. Jane Austen now has more posthumous diagnoses than novels. Cleared at last of Addison's disease, she has dusted off conjunctivitis, eczema and arthritis, enjoyed a brief flirtation with infectious mononucleosis from a stolen kiss before erupting into purpura, and written her last three novels secretly cherishing a Hodgkin's lymphoma which will eventually kill her.

Jane, with one scathing phrase, would have ditched these presumptions and settled for that cold. Colds, after all, were her most effective literary device. She used them with brilliant effect to precipitate ardour, unmask villainy and enforce propinquity to bring a simmering romance to the boil. Without a good cold, most of her novels would collapse.

Lacking her wit, I can only silently agree. One can die after catching a cold in 2020—especially in the cold.

Most colds are viral, and virologists have grouped the culprits by seasonality: those present throughout the year, those with winter preponderance, and those with a preference for warmer temperatures.

Where does SARS-CoV-2 fit in?

Respiratory infections are common in cold dry weather. And there are reasons enough:

~ Ciliary activity is poor at low temperatures, and the airway gets clogged with microbes that would otherwise be filtered out.

~ The respiratory lining becomes dry, and without the protection of mucus, it is an easy target for infections.

~ People stay home in a huddle, sharing each others' microbes and allowing infective strains to emerge through recombination.

~ Abrupt cooling results in the constriction of blood vessels in the upper airways. This can alter the inflammatory profile and change a latent (asymptomatic) infection into an overt illness.

But we don't really know, do we? Covid-19 has shown us there's a lot we can't explain about climate and viral emergence, virulence and our own immune response.

The commonest upper respiratory infections are caused by rhinoviruses; in a cold climate, signs of infection usually follow seventy-two hours after a recorded temperature and humidity decrease. Then come the coronaviruses which cause common colds. Do they follow a similar pattern? Does SARS-COV-2?

Wuhan had an average temperature of 8°C through December 2019, with a minimum of 0°C. It was foggy, most days the haze never lifted. Was the cold a driver for the emergence of Covid-19?

Silicosis is rampant in China, and the Hubei province is one of the worst affected regions. The disease profile has occupied Chinese experts for a long time, and industrial precautions are now the rule.

It isn't all about industrial exposure. Silicosis can be a silent presence in the lungs of people unconnected with the handling of stone materials, but who live in the vicinity of stone industries. The urban population of any large metropolis, and indeed members of a family where home remodelling and repairs involve drilling and polishing, are exposed to silica that can be inhaled. This inhaled silica is phagocytosed by alveolar cells. It engages in the pro-inflammatory cascade. It sets up chronic inflammation long before 'silicosis' is diagnosed on X-rays.

When I spoke with experts who recorded silicosis in agate workers of Khambat, I realised the protean character of the illness. Agate polishing is a familial skill. The stories of survivors are family histories. In two days of listening to survivors narrate horrendous stories of loss, I encountered not one but multiple diseases.

To agate workers, silicosis has a predictable profile. It begins with a cough that progresses to breathlessness. It limits activity and thrusts the young into an abrupt senescence. They lie wasted, bedridden, impatient for death. These workers were also familiar with a disease they called silicoTB—many lung pathologies, all caused by tuberculosis, coexisted with silicosis. Then, there was acute silicosis, recalled as 'sudden death'. In this, the pneumonia that swiftly led to fatal ARDS was so sudden in its onset, and killed so quickly, it almost erased itself.

A fourth category, which they did not connect with silicosis, was made of the multiple ailments they ascribed as the also-rans in their litany of woes—arthritis, kidney disease, recurrent skin afflictions. These suggested an autoimmune process was at work. A silica-injured lung has a defective immune response, which makes it susceptible to infection and autoimmune disease.

The airway lining is the fraught arena of host–virus interaction. Tolerance to the virus can be impaired by the innate immune response raised by environmental pollutants like silica. With special reference to Hubei, engineered nanomaterials from the electronics industry produce particulates that are strong irritants. Carbon nanotubes, for instance, can set up severe inflammation in the lungs.

Analysts are certain the epidemic in Wuhan retreated because severe measures of physical distancing and isolation were strictly enforced.

What if we look at this tangentially?

As noted before, after the lockdown, the improvement in Wuhan's AQI was dramatic. This would have cleared the air of major respiratory irritants. The air was back to what it was *before* December 2019, when the virus would have been inhaled and exhaled, as it probably has been for the past forty years—*without causing illness.*

Clearing the air of particulates immediately relieves the airway of pro-inflammatory overlay. This means: no alveolar injury, no severe pneumonia, no ARDS, no deaths.

If this theory holds true, it should reflect in the experience of other countries too.

Does it?

Iran and Italy had severe outbreaks very early in 2020.

Iran has a high incidence of silicosis, and most of its victims are miners and agate workers. The country has more than 5,000 mines, and many of these are open-pit silica mines. Not only does that mean intensive and prolonged exposure for those in the industry, but wind-borne silica could be inhaled over a very large perimeter, with people far removed from the industry at considerable risk.

Asbestos mining flourished in northern Italy till 1985. Presently, Italy has a thriving artificial stone industry. Artificial stone is made from finely pulverised stone mixed with a synthetic resin. Its silica content, as high as 90 per cent, makes it extremely hazardous. Asbestos was banned in 1992, and presently, very low occupational limits are in place for both asbestos and crystalline silica.

But silica in the lungs has very long latency. It is often detected decades after retirement from active exposure—those who were most affected by Covid-19 were aged eighty years or above.

The United States, with the highest number of ARDS deaths so far, bears a heavy load of silica that can be inhaled from fracking and ozone smog.

Compared to these countries, outstripping even China at its worst, is the air pollution in India. New Delhi today has an unbelievable AQI of 87, but 500+ was the norm throughout last winter. If suspended particulate matter is so vital a determinant of Covid-19, why is India's case-load relatively mild?

That puzzled me, and it still does. But a likely explanation stares us in the face if we refuse the Wuhan grid.

Factor II

Yes, the first outbreak of Covid-19 was reported from Wuhan, but that doesn't necessarily mean the virus emerged there, nor that it was the first instance of human infection.

Air travel has been used to explain the rapid appearance of infection the world over. Is it explanation enough? We're still only backtracking contacts, desperately trying to connect them to the only acknowledged source—Wuhan. What if there were other points of origin?

Though the date of a virus's emergence can be calculated genetically, RNA viruses have a high recombination rate, and this obfuscates calculations. Although we earlier presumed SARS-CoV-2 emerged in December 2019, new genomic studies suggest it emerged from the bat coronavirus RaTG13 forty to seventy years ago. RaTG13 is the closest bat lineage to SARS-CoV-2. A sub-lineage of this bat virus can infect humans. Two sister lineages to RTG13/SARS-CoV-2 infect pangolins.

It is likely there was a direct spillover from bats into humans.

This long period of quiescence suggests SARS-CoV-2 has been circulating innocuously in bats and intermediate hosts all this while. Has it been innocuously circulating in humans too?

What caused it to erupt now as a dangerous disease?

The SARS-CoV-2 genomes circulating as local infections have been compared with the reference genome released in early January, and the findings are very interesting. From February onwards, as local transmission was reported from most countries, point mutations have been found, distinct to geographic areas. Three recurrent mutations have been found in Europe, and three others in North America.

These have not been found in Asia. A mutation in the *RdRp* gene itself (position 14408) has been associated with the increasing number of point mutations in European genomes after 20 February 2020. This has led researchers to speculate if this mutation may have increased virulence and replication rates, given the seriousness of the outbreak after 20 February. Mutations in *RdRp* may also impact therapy, by making affected people resistant to a particular drug. It is possible that different therapies may suit different populations.

There's a marked genetic diversity among Indian SARS-CoV-2 isolates. Two clusters have been identified: one group synchronises with genomes from Oceania, South Asia and the Middle East, the other with genomes from Europe. These groups are further distinguished by different clades. The disease in India is still developing.

These mutations are only to be expected, and they have occurred locally.

SARS-CoV-2 is an RNA virus, after all.

It is of interest if the severity of disease is associated with these mutations.

I don't think they can be ascribed solely to Wuhan contacts. I expect, soon, to read evidence of the virus having been in circulation long before the Wuhan outbreak.

We are still connecting the dots, several months into the pandemic.

I believe Covid-19 has a multifocal emergence, through multiple spillovers.

Bats are everywhere. In many European countries, the use of bats for mosquito control became popular in the wake of Zika and quietly increased the human–chiropteran interface.

The explosive outbreaks in several countries—Iran, Italy, Ecuador, United States—have been ascribed to an 'imported infection' brought into these countries by travellers. Are these local eruptions evidence of spillovers?

The puzzle is—why? What are the environmental drivers that compel a spillover? Have bat habitats been disturbed? Has the human–chiropteran interface become more intimate? Have bats moved into urban spaces?

Or, have they acquired more convenient intermediate hosts?

Unless we consider these questions, we will persist in the self-defeating blockade of quarantine and isolation, attributing spread to human agency alone.

If we consider the possibility of multiple spillovers, we need more information about both reservoir and intermediate hosts.

Though it is being done, the viral sampling of bats is a tremendously difficult undertaking. When we consider the staggering numbers of viruses bats carry, their longevity, their vagility and the number of species they or their secretions encounter, the task seems impracticable. It is far easier to surveil the other end of the equation—us. The intelligent approach, rather, would be to become more aware of the bat–human interface.

For instance, the largest urban bat colony in North America is located in Austin, Texas, underneath the Ann W. Richards Congress Avenue bridge. One-and-a-half million bats reportedly live there. It is a virus hotspot. Do spillovers regularly occur there? Mapping such areas for known viral diseases would be illuminating. While this is an enormous colony, and therefore easily identified, smaller colonies should also be mapped as critical zones and the human–chiropteran interface restricted.

Multiple spillovers would also explain the rate of spread in different countries. India, with its population density, has had a very moderate profile. For India, lockdown has meant great hazards. The loss of income, shelter and food has forced migrant workers to move out of cities that will no longer support them, to seek their distant homes, which no longer welcome them, because the village dreads the virus the prodigal brings home. For those at home in cities, home is often a ten square foot space with ten inhabitants, no ventilation or running water, chancy electricity and barely enough food. It is a magnificent milieu to amplify infections. Add to this the crowds at food distributions, at railway stations, at truck stops, and we can expect a huge explosion of infections.

We aren't seeing that—not yet—but we may in the coming months. This isn't prediction. As summer advances, fruits ripen, bats increase around fruit trees…and so do people.

By the end of July we should have been asking:

How has the pandemic changed bat habitats?

Factor III

The emergence of Covid-19 eventually has to do with a host factor that seems the common denominator for its myriad manifestations—inflammation.

One of the increasingly noticed features of the disease is that the younger patients who develop ARDS are obese. The usual reason ascribed for this is that obesity is associated with poor lung expansion. But that is no more than the tip of the iceberg.

Visceral fat deposits, always increased in obesity, have a strong pro-inflammatory profile. Obesity is a state of chronic inflammation, and the engagement of ACE2 receptors by the virus enhance this, priming the body for a cytokine storm.

My counter-view shifts the attention from the virus to us.

Inhaled particulates PM2.5 injure the lung and maintain a state of chronic inflammation.

Our strategy against COVID-19 should first focus on improving air quality, as clearing the air may reduce the number of severe cases.

Addressing obesity is the second step.

The third is to respect bat habitats and to demarcate them as critical zones.

These are things we can do while we wait for intelligent therapies and a safe vaccine.

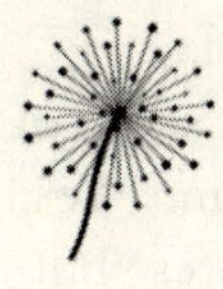

34

In India, Today

When we try to pick out anything by itself,
we find it hitched to everything else in the Universe.

– John Muir

By the time they're teenagers, most Indian children are anxious about just one acronym: NEET. The National Eligibility-cum-Entrance Test decides the fortunes of every student. Parental and peer pressure coupled with the arrant number in the competition place a cruel burden on young minds. Brilliant performers in the Board examinations find themselves out in the cold.

The NEET requires a score of over 600 out of 720 for eligibility to study medicine. Yes, private medical colleges will consider lower scores but at unaffordable prices. Medicine and engineering are still considered, by Indian parents, as the most stable and lucrative of career choices for their children.

The children, who may have a different opinion, are confronted with this unanswerable question: *What can you know of life at sixteen?*

The truth is, parents of forty know nothing at all about the life a sixteen-year-old will grow into. By the time these children are forty, doctors and engineers may be irrelevant—doctors already are, supplanted by the abler, if gnomic, internet.

Still, children disappointed by their NEET scores look around for alternatives, and for a decade now, the brightest on the horizon has been China.

China accepts students on the basis of Indian NEET scores, in fact welcomes those with scores of anything beyond 400. When I learnt of this, I remembered, with a smile, the college principal who had refused me admission.

'I won't take you because your marks are no good,' she said sternly. Then, she amended in a gentler voice, 'You're no good to us here.' She smiled at my indignant protest. 'We take students who have just scraped through school and make certain they graduate from here with honours. We don't need toppers like you.'

It took a long argument, but I stayed.

They don't make teachers like that in India any longer. Perhaps in China they do.

Certainly, the 2,000-odd Indian medical students currently training in China have felt welcome. Their parents, too, have an easier fee structure to deal with—on par with government or municipal colleges here, but way below what private colleges fleece you for. The instruction is in English, the campuses are comfortable and well equipped, the medical degree is recognised in India. What's not to like?

So, when Covid-19 broke out in Wuhan, there were a lot of Indian medical students there; Wuhan University regularly enrols international students. Most students were home on vacation, for the Chinese New Year, when Covid-19 erupted. Others managed to get away just before the lockdown was announced on 23 January.

Among the students who returned home to Kerala, one tested positive. He is among the first three cases reported in India, all from Kerala.

The index case in any epidemic is usually honoured by name. But like the three index cases in China, India's too is unnamed. He is a twenty-three-year-old medical student, and I wonder if he knows he has a place in history.

His five-day itinerary from Wuhan to Kasargod in Kerala is complicated:

22 January: Leaves Wuhan University for Guangzhou.

23 January–25 January: Spends time with friends in Guangzhou.

25 January: Flies to Kolkata, and thence to Bengaluru, where he stays overnight in a hotel.

26 January: Takes a flight to Cochin. Then a taxi from Cochin airport to Aluva railway station for the train to Kasargod. Discovering there's no sleeping berth available, he breaks his journey at Angamaly, where he stays overnight.

27 January: Takes a taxi to Angamaly station, and boards a train to Kanhangad. At Kanhangad, he shares a taxi with two others to arrive in Kasargod at dusk.

28 January: Reports to the district Corona Control Centre.

30 January: Develops a mild respiratory infection.

31 January: Gets admitted to the district hospital.

He has nothing worse than a cold and slightly sore throat. His physical parameters are normal. He tests positive for SARS-CoV-2 on RT-PCR. After several throat swabs are negative, he is released from hospital on 16 February. For the next twelve days, he is home quarantined. (The word 'strict' qualifies all directives.) He is finally declared harmless to the public on 28 February.

Much ado about nothing?

Not if we look at the Indian picture today as consequent to longitudinal transmission from a Wuhan import. In that case, every containment measure was justly and effectively applied.

Contact tracing was also set up immediately. His itinerary makes for tedious reading—but I have put it in to illustrate the magnitude of contact tracing. The number was fixed at

189 primary contacts and 305 secondary ones—a cheerily optimistic estimate, but one has to cap it somewhere.

The traced contacts were monitored for symptoms, and a few of them were tested too. They all tested negative.

Thus ended, happily, the successful containment of India's first import of Covid-19.

But by then, 28 February, India was already in panic.

The early response consisted of curtailing entry into the country and surveillance at airports. Testing was confined to those who had travelled internationally and were now experiencing symptoms of fever and cough, and for health workers in contact with patients with severe respiratory illness from any cause. By 28 February, 362 nasopharyngeal swabs from travellers were tested for a wide range of respiratory viruses, in addition to SARS-CoV-2.

One-fourth were positive for other respiratory viruses. Four were positive for SARS-CoV-2—three samples were from Kerala (including our medical student), and one from Delhi. Between 22 January to 29 February, there were no further positives for SARS-CoV-2.

These initial observations were limited to 'imports' from other countries.

India's first Covid-19 death was recorded on 13 March. Until that Friday, the Central government did not acknowledge a national health crisis. There were no restrictions in place, and no rules for public precautionary measures.

Beginning on 17 March, international travellers were home quarantined. During this period, two large 'imports' occurred. One was the Italian cluster that has by now passed out of national memory.

The second was the Tablighi Jamaat cluster that fed into the communal hatred that has destroyed our nation since

1992. It aroused the basest and most barbaric responses to suffering by criminalising the disease. North India projected hate at its inhuman worst, going to excesses that can only be termed psychopathic, and do not bear recall. This caused more suffering than any virus ever can. It was, truly, the darkest and most shameful moment in India's Covid-19 story.

Both clusters have relevance to the ideas in this book.

The Italian cluster can be traced back to 21 February, when twenty-three Italian tourists arrived in Delhi. Their group travelled in a coach with three Indians. The group included a doctor from Lombardy who, two days into the trip, developed fever, cough and breathlessness, but continued his tour. On 28 February, while touring Rajasthan, he was hospitalised with pneumonia. He was found to be Covid-19 positive, after which he was isolated in Jaipur. His wife, who also tested positive, was isolated with him. The other twenty-four members of the group, twenty-one Italians and three Indians, all asymptomatic, returned to Delhi on 2 March. They were all quarantined.

Out of this group, fifteen tested positive besides the sick doctor and his wife.

That is a very high 'attack rate'—65.4 per cent—compared with the national attack rate of 0.00332 per cent, which translates to only 33.2 people per million population.

This story ends badly, with two deaths.

It is important to all of us because it illustrates how proximity—and *enforced* proximity—increases infectivity. The closer we are packed together, the greater the chance of infection, and the greater too the virulence of the infection.

The Tablighi Jamaat congregation took place between 8 and 15 March in Delhi's Nizamuddin Markaz Masjid, near the famous shrine of Khwaja Nizamuddin Auliya. More than 9,000 missionaries attended this event. Besides those from different Indian states, there were international attendees.

On 16 March, a government order prohibited congregations of more than fifty people. On that day, ten Indonesians who had participated in the event in Delhi were isolated in Hyderabad. Seven tested positive. This set off contact tracing.

Following the imposition of the lockdown on 23 March, members of the Tablighi Jamaat were asked to evacuate the building, tested and quarantined. By this time, many had travelled home. In the following weeks, we witnessed the dragnet of contact tracing across the nation.

As clusters announced themselves across states, by 3 April, 647 of the total 664 cases were linked to this event.

As the news spread, so did the hate. The 'investigation' abandoned all semblance of science. It became a witch hunt, on social media and on the street.

This event showed, yet again, what is driving this pandemic in India—human density.

The population density in India is 464 people per square kilometre, calculated on a total land area of 2,973,190 square kilometres.[18]

The average Indian household has three to four members living in a 10'x10' space. Compound this with the miseries of lockdown, where large numbers have been constrained into small spaces. You need only walk through a Mumbai slum or a Delhi jhuggee to understand this. It cannot be imagined. Nor can you grasp what it means to live like that unless you do so yourself. It takes as much intelligence as

---

18. Worldometer, 2020. https://www.worldometers.info/world-population/india-population/.

endurance to weather, negotiate and navigate your way out into the world.

'These days you can never tell. These girls look so smart you'd never guess they came from a slum.' This appalling remark to me came from a 'respected' senior journalist.

The man's soul stank, and I've avoided him since.

But the statement is a succinct précis of the caste system. Blindness, obliteration, outrage and resentment—delivered in one neat phrase of condescension and patronage.

Within hours of the lockdown, as businesses downed shutters, millions were stranded without jobs. This meant, very quickly, no shelter and no food.

There was only one place to go—home.

Home was more a destination of the spirit, despite its geographic location. The only thing that mattered was the getting there.

People moved, no matter how. They walked, hitched rides or cycled. Starved and dehydrated, exhausted to the point of collapse, they reached home at last, to sullen indifference, rejection or despair.

Where will they go from here? To many, the only answer is to trek back to their old jobs. But will those jobs be waiting for them? Uncertainty, dread and hunger loom. If they contract Covid-19, what chance do they have of survival?

Every Indian city is powered by these men and women, most of them young. When the lockdown was announced, why was their existence not noticed? They aren't migrants, as a journalist observed angrily; they are Indians, like you or me.

How astute was her comment. One doesn't migrate within one's own country; one belongs.

Overlooking, ignoring, obliterating the summarily disempowered has criminalised them. They are now seen as vectors of disease.

A lockdown is excellent epidemiological control on paper. It reduces the number of contacts dramatically. It reduces the viral load in inhaled air. By shutting down vehicular traffic and industries, it reduces particulate matter in the air.

It is the ideal epidemiological response in a wealthy country with excellent infrastructure and a small population that can retire into comfortable bunkers, country homes, dachas—assured of being supplied all they demand, confident of space and ease and communication, trusting in a stable healthcare system and assured of social security.

Yes, a lockdown will then definitely 'flatten the curve'. We've seen that happen, with relief and hope, in European countries.

But the realities of poorer nations like India, Bangladesh, Brazil, Pakistan, Peru and the Philippines are very different.

At the beginning of the lockdown on 23 March, India had nine deaths from Covid-19. The squeeze of the past months has crowded people into small spaces (their homes)—or large public spaces, like Shramik trains.

By 23 April, there were 681 Covid-19 deaths.

By 23 May, 3,720 deaths.

By 15 June, 8,884 deaths, with 396 deaths every day.

And now, as you read this, how many have died since then?

Testing is restricted to very few, so the number of 'active' or 'positive' cases has no meaning. By now, the virus is everywhere. It is the deaths we must go by. And the facts are unarguable: the disease has increased in virulence.

Earlier, there was a great deal of talk about 'immunity' in Indians that protected us from the worst of Covid-19. Needless to say, such beliefs came packaged with hoary traditions: go-mutra and turmeric vied with Ganga-jal and superior genes. It is necessary to dismiss such tosh before we can explore the observation.

Since the Wuhan outbreak, SARS-CoV-2 has had several months to adapt and regroup its genes. It inhabits all of the planet now, including the poles. It has manifested differently in different countries. What does geography have to do with that?

Geography is history.

Geneticists have studied genomes of the virus from different countries and examined emerging mutations. Have these mutations increased the virulence of the disease?

The virus has spread more rapidly since March. There is now a larger database available for analysis from different geographic regions. It is evident that SARS-CoV-2 has undergone many mutations. This highlights the observation that local varieties replace the parent strain of virus. To me, this also suggests the possibility of multiple spillovers.

India may be late in exhibiting its particular genetic type. As the spillover from bats coincides with the fruiting season, an increase of cases through June to August might establish an Indian 'type'.

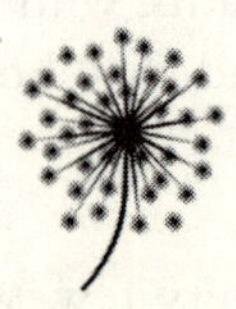

35

'Please Scream Within Your Heart'

The past is the present, isn't it? It's the future, too.
We all try to lie out of that but life won't let us.

– Eugene O'Neill, *Long Day's Journey into Night*, 1941

If SARS-CoV-2 is shed with each exhalation, what's the etiquette for joy? For anguished abandon? For discomfiture? How to contain the moment's urgency?

Fuji-Q Highland Amusement Park advises riders on roller coasters to *'Please Scream Within Your Heart'*.

Rachel Carson should have called her book *Silent Scream.*

Several months into the pandemic, we must refuse this silence and give vent to the scream locked deep in our hearts.

This is the silence of rage, not helplessness.

It is the soundless implosion of truth.

A succinct elucidation appeared in *The Indian Express* on 6 July. From Sultanganj of Bhagalpur district in Bihar, journalist Dipankar Ghose reported the effects of lockdown on school children deprived of the mid-day school meal:

> 'Haan' (yes) they shout when asked if they got food in school.
>
> 'Nahin' (no) they say, more quietly, when asked if they have any food during the day, now that schools are shut.
>
> And what was their favourite day in school?
>
> 'Friday' they shout, the one day in the week when eggs were served.

This is what COVID-19 has accomplished. But seriously, should we blame the virus for this heinous crime? This is the reality of India, a country polarised between want and excess.

At six months, humanity took stock of the pandemic: on 1 July, the WHO had recorded 10.36 million cases and 508,055 deaths worldwide.

The biggest worry isn't the rising death rate but the number of infected people who are asymptomatic. They make up more than 40 per cent of the infected and, unless tested, cannot be identified, remaining potential sources of infection. Most quickly test negative on PCR, much quicker than people with even mild symptoms.

An allied worry is people who continue to test positive on nasopharyngeal swabs long after they have recovered.

Where is the virus hiding?

Think back to the early part of this book, where we spoke about the airway. The paranasal sinuses, lined with velvety mucosa, are rich in ACE2 receptors and are a refuge for inhaled viruses. Mucosal linings have local immune systems, and these may be important sites for determining infectivity and deciding viral shedding. Doctors who deal with the upper airway—ENT surgeons, anaesthetists and dentists—are exposed to the highest possible viral load when they deal with infected patients.

What have we learnt about the disease process in COVID-19? This is vital. It will advise our approach in the days ahead.

We have moved to a better understanding of what this virus targets.

SARS-Co-V-2 appears to fixate on the endothelium, the specialised inner lining of blood vessels.

COVID-19 patients at grave risk are those with extant endothelial disease. Co-morbidities—obesity, hypertension, diabetes—all affect the endothelium. As illness worsens, disorders of blood clotting and inflammation of blood vessels, manifest as complications. This tells us the primary site of affliction is the endothelium. It also explains the wide-spread destruction of organ tissue which culminates in multi-organ failure.

The earliest reports of COVID-19 demonstrated the profile of uncontrolled, uncontrollable, inflammation. We discussed this at length. Endothelial cells are more than just blood vessel lingerie. They regulate blood flow and blood pressure and secrete chemicals that affect the organs around them.

Remember the inflammatory molecule IL-6, which we met early in this book? IL-6 induces endothelial cells to secrete pro-inflammatory cytokines. Not only does it contribute to the inflammatory process, it also alters the functions of the endothelial cells. They can no longer regulate clotting factors in the blood. Tiny clots, microthrombi, form as a consequence and damage vital organs. Larger clots, especially in the blood vessels of the lung, can lead to rapid worsening of health and sudden death.

Presently, a lot of research is directed at the role of the endothelial cell in COVID-19, studying its direct engagement with the virus and its response to inflammatory cytokines like IL-6. The success of tocilizumab, an IL-6 blocker, is probably because it preserves endothelial cell function.

What have we learnt about spread?

Quite a lot, it appears, and conversely, nothing at all.

It grows more evident each day that this virus is airborne. Being airborne means a greater ambit: the virus can be dispersed widely from ventilation ducts and air conditioners. Indeed, from speech, laughter, cough, and the simple act of easy exhalation.

How do we counter it?

We have been doing so for centuries.

Leave your windows open.

By now, surely, the virus is everywhere. Time we put an end to our ostrich act of isolation?

We should take heart from the discovery that SARS-CoV-2 isn't very viable on surfaces—can we *please* ease up on drenching the planet in disinfectant?

We have more evidence of how the outcome in COVID-19 is decided not by the virus but by us.

A recent report estimated that one in five individuals worldwide is at increased risk of developing severe disease if infected, *because of an underlying condition*. The study calculates the risk at less than 5 per cent in those younger than 20 years to more than 66 per cent in those 70 years or older.

It echoes the thought that fills this book: if you have an illness that puts you at risk, get medical attention now.

Quite at variance with this advice is the most serious consequence of this pandemic: the neglect of other illnesses, especially in children who are missing out on immunisations and food.

Diphtheria has resurfaced in Pakistan, Nepal and Bangladesh. A newly mutated version of poliovirus has begun a slow but certain globe trot. Cholera outbreaks have been reported in Bangladesh, Yemen, Cameroon, Mozambique and South Sudan. Measles, almost forgotten as a childhood killer, is re-emerging everywhere.

This reappearance of childhood diseases reveals the shameful callousness of our species. Is it not a biological imperative to protect our children?

Early in this pandemic, the all-absorbing question was not whether COVID-19 infected children or the unborn, it was *whether children could spread the disease.* Yes, there was a rationale to this. Still, it was a chilling inversion of the biological impulse.

Children are no longer considered safe from COVID-19. Not after childhood multi-system inflammatory syndrome (MIS-C) is being reported from every affected country.

This condition is encountered in children who have not suffered clinical disease, but have been exposed to infected adults. Some of these children have recovered from a mild infection. MIS-C develops about three weeks after such a history. It can be overwhelmingly sudden or begin insidiously, with fever and diarrhoea.

Initially, we read about this development in anecdotes describing different symptoms. It took a while to realise we were looking at different facets of a new, peculiar manifestation of COVID-19. The press went to town and called it Kawasaki disease. That's inaccurate.

MIS-C occurs two to four weeks after infection or contact. The virus may be detected on PCR or antibodies to the virus may be present in the child. It is more common among Asians, African-Americans and Hispanics. I worry about what could happen in India and Africa.

As the name suggests, it is a multi-organ disease that quickly makes a child critically ill. Cardiac complications are common and early.

Most children will recover. But why should they get ill at all?

Emerging research points to disordered immunity

yet again—this time, the cells responsible for adaptive immunity.

Life, for us, has certainly changed.

But how have the past months changed the virus?

Changes in the behaviour of a virus come from mutations, which usually confer an advantage to the virus.

One such mutation of SARS-CoV-2 was identified in February. This mutation is not observed in other coronaviruses that use the ACE2 receptor, so it may have emerged to compensate for the newly acquired furin site that cleaves the S1-S2 spike protein in SARS-Co-V2. This mutation, called D614G, began spreading in Europe in early February. Soon, it dominated the Covid landscape in every new outbreak.

In addition, there is evidence that the virus undergoes recombination with local strains. This raises, again, the possibility of multiple spillovers. I strongly feel that tracing the emergence of new strains of SARS-CoV-2 in parallel with bat behaviour will help map the progress of Covid-19 in a more practical and controllable manner.

Evidence of local infections of Covid-19 unrelated to Wuhan is increasing. The story of those Italian tourists in India has an interesting feature. The first person to fall ill, a doctor, was symptomatic when he arrived in India. This means he had been infected at least a week prior, perhaps by one of his patients. That was the time when sporadic cases began to be noticed in northern Italy.

A great deal of contact tracing was done to connect these cases with Wuhan, but it all seemed very deterministic to me.

Now, of course, we know.

The virus was being actively shed by Italians as long back as December 2019. Their sewage proves it: Italy's National Institute of Health announced, on 18 June, that sewage water samples of 18 December from Milan and Turin contained genetic traces of SARS-CoV-2.

It is time to rethink Covid-19. No more can we consider it as something that travelled in a straight line out from Wuhan.

Think of it as autochthonous, existing in nature—not just in the bat but in one or innumerable intermediate hosts.

Think of it as disinclined to spill over, unless we push it over the brink by felling trees, despoiling hillsides, disturbing caves.

Think of Covid-19 not as a killer disease but as an infection your body can resist. So start getting fit to counter it. If age isn't on your side, take shelter, but remember the ageing body has its own resources and can still put up a fight and win.

Above all, think of Covid-19 as part of the filthy air we breathe. Cleaner air will have fewer viruses, and our lungs will breathe more healthily.

All these months into the pandemic, it will be self-destructive to read it as a death warrant.

It is, in fact, a reprieve from certain disaster. A reminder to live as a sapient species again.

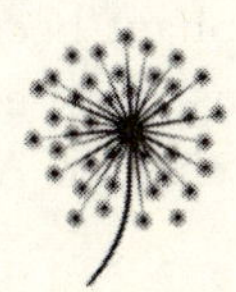

36

Do Elephants Get the Flu?

...the Universe is not only queerer than we suppose,
but queerer than we can suppose.
– J.B.S. Haldane, *Possible Worlds and Other Essays*, 1927

Do elephants get the flu? Do they get COVID-19? If I were to tell you that wild elephants in Botswana are dying mysteriously, would it worry you?

It worries me deeply. I worry that we have, in some unknown way, transmitted an illness to them.

You may disagree because, like the experts in Botswana, you know all about how those 400 elephants buckled at the knees after running around in circles and collapsed at the edge of a water-hole. That isn't COVID-19—we know from wisdom acquired through months of education in viruses, pandemics and isolation.

Or is it?

If we read the notes on patients with neurological fallout from COVID-19, we might spare a thought for those elephants.

We may be wrong. Sorry, *I* may be wrong.

Perhaps the tragic aerial photographs simply startled me.

We notice a dead elephant because when something as monolithic, as humungous as an elephant is stopped in its tracks, the elements are shaken. As they never are by the death of a fly.

Sizeism is another of our prejudices. Elephants don't share it. Nor do flies.

We haven't the vaguest idea what they think of us.

But then, they don't think. *We* are the intelligent species, remember?

Shouldn't we get intelligent about how Covid-19 has changed the wild?

Anecdotes blink in and promptly blink out on social media: bird sightings, tiny furry mammals cozying up trustingly, unexpected butterflies, mountain goats strolling through Welsh villages, bears checking out pubs. Adits for a new treasury of nursery literature.

But reality is grimmer.

Covid-19 might have thrust wildlife trade into the sun, but it hasn't curtailed it. The pangolin, poor mammal, is still avidly hunted. As smuggling routes are exposed and contraband animals, confined under unspeakable conditions, are shunted across borders and continents, the debate has shifted to whether they shed SARS-CoV-2 along the way.

What of the animals? Pangolin scutes are recovered by the ton in police raids. How many pangolins make 22 tons of scales?

Now that surveillance in Asia has doubled, the network has simply shifted to Africa. Rhino and elephant poaching is rampant. Bushmeat demand has increased. To humans, these changes present the threat of more zoönoses, many from unknown organisms.

India has a well documented history of zoönotic emergence in Kyasanur Forest disease, a hemorrhagic fever caused by a flavivirus that circulates among monkeys. The virus is transmitted by ticks. In 1957, dead monkeys were discovered when land was cleared for agriculture in Karnataka's Shimoga district. Soon, the illness was noticed in villages around the forest. This virus also circulates in birds, rodents and shrews and is no longer confined to Kyasanur. Cases have been reported in Gujarat, West Bengal, Andaman and Nicobar Islands.

Despite this understanding of how zoönoses develop and travel, we continue to ravage our forests. In India, only 4.9 per cent of land is protected for wildlife. These zones are home to 91,200 species of animals. That is 7.6 per cent of known mammalian, 12.6 per cent of avian and 6.2 per cent of reptilian species. All these small sanctuaries are battered by human encroachments.

The wild can be infected by diseases in livestock. Tuberculosis and brucellosis are well-known examples of this. Avian flu, the highly infectious poultry disease, is another. During a recent outbreak among domestic fowl in Assam, the virus was isolated from a jungle crow as well.

Japanese encephalitis is heartbreakingly common among inner-city Indian children. It is maintained in circulation by small water birds, egrets and herons that hover around pavement 'wet markets' in every city.

The human-wild interface is ubiquitous and unavoidable.

It isn't human disease but human health that is a mystery to me. After all the wrong we do, how does the world remain so right?

Covid-19 is not the last pandemic we will face, so we cannot afford to ignore any of its fallouts. Its impact on non-human life may ignite more zoönoses in future. Will that dread make our anthropocentric thinking a little more lateral?

Domestic animals, particularly cats, are susceptible to Covid-19. Will it spread, through one or many intermediate hosts, into the wild?

Do elephants get the flu?

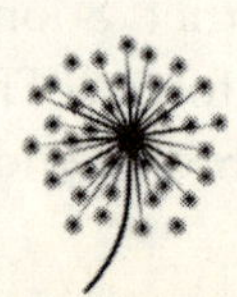

37

Testing, Therapy, Vaccine

The last capitalist we hang shall be the one
who sold us the rope.

– attributed to Vladimir Ilyich Lenin

'Christopher Columbus! What's the matter?' cried Jo, as Beth put out her hand as if to warn her off, and asked quickly…

'You've had the scarlet fever, haven't you?'

'Years ago, when Meg did. Why?'

'Then I'll tell you. Oh, Jo, the baby's dead!'

'What baby?'

'Mrs Hummel's. It died in my lap before she got home,' cried Beth with a sob.

We know how that turned out. Thanks to Greta Gerwig's brilliant film, *Little Women* has dusted off its cobwebs and is back in bookshops and libraries. And in the time of Covid-19, the travails of the March sisters have special resonance.

I was eight when the March girls introduced me to immunology. As the pages blurred through my tears, my vaccination scars throbbed with guilt. If only I had a vaccine, I could save Beth. What if—

'Nobody gets scarlet fever any more,' the doctor said shortly, shooing me out of his room.

Oh, but they do, I could have told him ten years later, when I met kids crippled with all the complications of a strep throat: endocarditis, rheumatic fever, nephritis.

In Louisa May Alcott's time, scarlet fever killed more children than Covid-19 has to date. The discipline then was no different from ours in this pandemic. The March girls had isolated themselves, and Beth recovered. But I hadn't, a year later, when I discovered scarlatina's treachery—the stuffy sequel, *Good Wives*, kills off Beth, by then the only decent girl left of the lot.

Our strongest, most universal, response to COVID-19 came out of *Little Women*. Since 1868, the book has never been out of print.

As a young girl, Alice Hamilton must have wept over it. As a medical student, Alice met scarlatina's germ, the streptococcus. In 1905, her observations were surprisingly given an airing in the very misogynistic world of medicine. Her paper 'Dissemination of Streptoccal Sputum', which appeared in the *Journal of the American Medical Association*, urged the absolute necessity of donning a mask in the presence of an infectious throat disease.

Masks were not unknown in 1905. They were sporadically used by surgeons. Jan Mikulicz-Radecki, the brilliantly innovative Polish surgeon, never operated without one. But though the German bacteriologist Carl Flügge had demonstrated, in the final decade of the nineteenth century, that exhaled air contained microbe-laden droplets,[19] these observations were dismissed as irrelevant to practice. Alice Hamilton didn't think so. She related the spread of the disease to droplet infection, and strongly advocated the use of masks in the operating room and while handling dressing materials.

Alice Hamilton, through 101 inspiring years, made many spectacular contributions to science. Medicine acknowledges

---

19. Even during 'quiet speech', minute droplets are sprayed in the air. These are called 'Flügge droplets' in honour of Carl Georg Friedrich Wilhelm Flügge, to give him his full name. He is best remembered for *Lehrbuch der Hygienischen Untersuchungsmethoden* (Textbook of Hygienic Investigation Methods).

a multiplicity of fathers for various skills and specialities, but no mothers. Hamilton was the 'mother of industrial medicine'. Her clear vision and remarkable intelligence brought to light innumerable instances of occupational hazards in factories and in the indeterminate use of fuels. In all that grand panorama of achievements, her paper on the necessity of surgical masks is a very small element, easily overlooked. But it has saved millions from surgical infections.

Will the mask save millions from COVID-19 too?

A recent paper from China recommends masking within the home, as most COVID-19 infections are from household transmission. To me, that's the ultimate alienation, but I won't be surprised if I'm the only one to think so. After all, COVID-19 isn't a missile with a mere six-foot range.

Looking closer at the way COVID-19 travels may be the right way to stop its spread. It is propelled out of the respiratory tract on a little hot cloud of turbulence that will waft it way beyond six feet.

Droplets are sized between ten to five microns. Aerosols are smaller than five-micron particles. Being lighter, they stay afloat longer. New measures of COVID-19 control, brace yourselves, might be directed against airborne aerosols, rather than droplet transmission.

Forget coughing or sneezing, aerosols are being blamed on breathing. Anything above a whisper, speech with more palatals and fewer fricatives, not to mention singing—they all charge the atmosphere thick with aerosols. Even quiet breathing, apparently, fills the air with contagion.

To be perfectly safe, neither an exhaler nor an inhaler be.

Seriously, *dead*?

The facts are indisputable, but come on, this is a respiratory virus. Where else, and how else, will it thrive except in humid propinquities?

WHO's early protocol on restricting the use of masks in Covid-19 to front-line workers and care-givers, we now learn, are from the 1930s, when, presumably, it was still legal to breathe. In the 1930s, the world had fresh in its memory a disaster far worse than Covid-19. It is worthwhile returning to early descriptions of the 1918 pandemic of influenza. If those directives worked then, they're still good to go.

Worthwhile too, while we consider droplets and aerosols, to remember the pneumonic plague of 1910 and the brilliant observations of the Malaysian doctor Wu Lien Teh in Manchuria.

His notes document how human-to-human transmission quickly established pneumonic plague:

> During our stay at Hailar, we noticed the gradual evolution of the plague from the bubonic through the septicaemic into the pneumonic form, due principally to promiscuous spitting and huddling together of coolies day and night in unventilated inns.

This is of great relevance to India, where lockdown has colluded with poverty in driving migrants to desperate measures. The trains deployed for their 'relief' are nothing short of death traps. What new manifestations of Covid-19 will be visited on the population as a result of such human suffering in enforced congestion? In any infection it is population density that decides the death toll.

Incidentally, Wu Lien Teh was also a pioneer in two other forms of containment that challenge us today. In 1910, he reached Harbin to investigate a killer disease that had practically wiped out the town. The streets of Harbin were piled with corpses, perfectly preserved in sub-zero temperatures that made it impossible to dig the ground for burial. The first post-mortem examination he conducted convinced him that this was a new sort of plague.

It might have been new to him, but not to Bombay, where, in 1896, bubonic plague had swiftly assumed killer avatars, like this one. Harbin had pneumonic plague, transmitted through inhalation.

Lien Teh isolated the plague bacillus from the lungs. His first act thereafter was to design a suitable mask, using several layers of surgical gauze. He employed everyone he knew in the urgent manufacture of masks, which he distributed all over Harbin.

This made him a laughing stock among his European colleagues. Gerald Mesny, a prominent French physician, cut a swagger through the plague-ridden town, sneering at Lien Teh's insistence on masks. Mesny died the next day of pneumonic plague.

Despite Lien Teh's efforts, the plague continued in Manchuria. It took Lien Teh a long while to notice the reason hiding in plain sight: the piles of corpses that jammed every street teemed with active bacilli. He lobbied for permission for a mass cremation, and finally got it. Once Harbin was rid of the infective corpses, cases of plague quickly diminished. The epidemic stopped.

In the Bombay plague, terribly mismanaged though it was, clear rules were laid down for disposal of the dead early in the epidemic.

In India today, such rules have yet to trickle down to public consciousness. The press reports shocking incidents of relatives refusing to accept bodies, of public outrages at funerals. The decencies of last rites are repudiated.

Such shameful cruelties are the responses of a panicked population.

As of now, Covid-19 has neither treatment nor vaccine. The only method available to arrest its spread is to identify the vulnerable and isolate them from the source of infection.

Who is the source of infection? Who is vulnerable?

Everyone.

A person infected with Covid-19 is most infectious *before* he falls sick. Just about anyone could be coughing, sneezing, or simply exhaling the virus.

All 7.8 billion of us are exposed to factors that maim the lung. All of us are vulnerable.

The only logical solution, which is to isolate ourselves from each other, is sheer lunacy. Saner far to identify both groups: the infectious by wide testing, and the vulnerable by identifying the risk factors and addressing them.

Till we do that, we are stuck in this apausalypse, panicked ostriches, heads buried deep in the sand.

What happens when we pull out of our lockdowns? The enemy is still here, isn't it?

Epidemiology tells us that it is in the nature of epidemics to peter out once a population is immune.

Such general truths no longer apply. These ideas are in continuum with an older view of disease emergence and spread.

Novel viruses don't seem to conform to this. MERS-CoV is still in circulation, eight years after it emerged.

There is no sign of herd immunity to Covid-19, several months into the pandemic.

As we have to rely completely on non-pharmacological methods, we had better rethink strategy. If we want to put an end to this pandemic, we must stop looking at mathematical curves and start looking at people.

Containment and mitigation are big words. Containing the pandemic has no meaning if it does not mitigate human suffering. Since wide testing has been possible in very few countries, the 'number of cases' is actually a misnomer. It is more honest to first state the number of people actually tested before stating the number that tested positive.

'Spread' is not a territorial advancement. It is the transfer of virus from one human being to another. It might work in mathematics to believe that the increasing number of deaths can be reconciled with a containment plan, but not in reality.

Covid-19 is not a graph. It is your life and mine on the line.

Tests are expensive, but governments have to afford them. They must be made free of charge.

We only have one reliable test at the moment—the RT-PCR, which detects viral particles. It is usually tested on nasopharyngeal swabs. In hospitalised patients who are severely ill and intubated, the test can done on deeper respiratory secretions.

People exposed to an infected person must be tested five days after contact. Earlier testing may be negative. Tests are also needed to declare a patient disease-free. Two 'negatives' spaced forty-eight hours apart are generally taken as sufficient evidence of cure. Testing stool samples may be a better idea. The virus continues to be shed in stool days after it has disappeared from the respiratory tract.

Moreover, antibody tests are iffy. Many patients do not show seropositivity despite having the disease. That apart, the test itself does not have convincing reliability. Many countries have used pulse oximetry as a screening tool in patients who are 'apparently normal' but show signs of developing pneumonia on X-ray or CT scans—a drop in blood oxygenation is considered an alarm signal.

I want to mention a non-pharmacological treatment that is of great value even in critical patients. It is the simple measure of 'proning'—lying on the stomach (or on the side for the obese patient). This change of posture improves oxygenation. It is being used with success in patients with early respiratory failure.

Drugs for Covid-19 are being designed with these targets in view:

1. The engagement between the spike protein and the ACE2 receptor,
2. The fusion of the spike protein with the cell membrane,
3. The replication of the virus,
4. The inflammatory response.

The oldest drug in use is the trusted antimalarial chloroquine and its congener hydroxychloroquin. Initial enthusiasm for these drugs, which act as antivirals and immuno-modulators, has worn off after reports of adverse effects such as sudden cardiac crises.

After the international controversy over disturbing results, WHO has withdrawn them. Inexplicably, they continue to be used in India, justified by that irrefutable argument: 'We've used it for ages as malaria prophylaxis, so it can't hurt now.' Again, for some of us, progress is the reassessment of 'experience'.

The antiviral drug remdesivir disables the viral replicase gene and stops virus replication.

The interleukin-antagonist anakinra, trialled in COVID-19 patients with mild ARDS and hyper-inflammation, shows promise.

Cytokine storm, the fatal event in COVID-19, is the focus of attention. Interleukin blockers like tocilizumab are being used.

A number of treatment options are being talked about.

Do they work?

Are they dangerous?

When should they be administered?

Can they be used to prevent the worst of the illness?

These are nightmare questions for both doctor and patient.

And these are the only two people who matter, for even a pandemic is reduced to one patient's experience.

And that experience is a relationship, albeit very brief, between two consenting individuals.

Eventually, the doctor will make the decision and choose the drug that best serves the moment.

True, there are treatment protocols, but often the attending physician has to step across those boundaries and fall back on her own intelligence, training and experience.

Vaccines?

A safe vaccine is at least a year away.

Till then, why not rely on our ability to stave off disease?

The neglected factor in the world's COVID-19 strategy is—you.

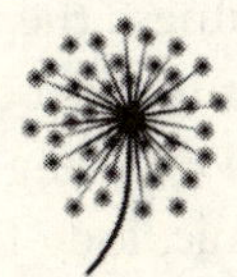

38
Primum Non Nocere

For I have learned
To look on nature, not as in the hour
Of thoughtless youth; but hearing oftentimes
The still, sad music of humanity
– William Wordsworth, 'Lines Composed a Few Miles above Tintern Abbey, On Revisiting the Banks of the Wye during a Tour', 13 July 1798

The literature of plagues fills libraries. Most accounts relate to *the* plague, oracular now and of great historic value. But what did they mean to their authors, these lines of reportage, lamentation, despair?

The act of writing was everything. It was duty, not self-indulgence. Those chroniclers wrote because the moment demanded it. They merely succumbed to the urgency even the humblest hack knows: the need to inscribe—on clay, on stone, on palm leaf, papyrus, parchment, paper, or even the ephemeral computer screen.

It is what we do.

The compulsion that produces graffiti on the toilet wall is no different from what drove Thucydides to take notes on the Athenian plague. *Kilroy was here* is much older than the Second World War. It predates language, perhaps even sentience, this need to witness the moment.

It compelled me to write this book, knowing as I did the danger of writing into an evolving story. I began this book very early into the epidemic, long before the WHO granted it pandemic status on 11 March.

Covid-19 unfurled like an invisible *Rafflesia* bloom: no root nor stem nor leaf, recognisable only from the miasma of death it left downwind. I was its companion, hamsafar, through its puzzling masquerade. It unmasked often, and each time revealed a different face.

From being a purely respiratory disease in December 2019, it has widened into one with neurological, cardiovascular and renal complications. The only clue of its presence may be gastrointestinal. It can affect infants and toddlers. It can devastate children with a mysterious multi-organ inflammation. It can still the heart, while mild in its other afflictions. And it can do all this after it declares itself gone with a mocking negative RT-PCR result.

So far, there is no news of sexual transmission, nor of the virus crossing the placenta—but who can tell?

I expect it to act out the myth of Raktabīja, a new form springing up at every new outbreak. My gut feeling is that even with 10.19 million confirmed cases and 503,862 deaths (according to the WHO Covid-19 Situation Report for 30 June), it is only Act I of this tragedy.

Writing this book has been a race to keep abreast and analyse information as it emerged these past months. Every line was written with a curious fatalism that it would have to be erased the next week. There is every chance that by this time next year this book will need revision. Discovery is always just round the corner.

A few years ago, I wrote a book about Bombay's Gilbert Hill. Four years of practically camping on site—photographing the hill from every angle, through sun and wind and rain, delving cross-eyed through old maps, plans and manuscripts—got me nowhere towards discovering the eponymous Gilbert. I shamefacedly had to acknowledge the lacuna. Two years later, while researching the Bombay plague, whom do I meet but Mr Gilbert! He is still waiting, impatiently, to reclaim his Hill, but I've lost all hope of seeing him in a new edition of *Once Upon a Hill.* Meanwhile, the hill has been reduced to a bump in the Sierra Nueva of concrete replicating faster than SARS-CoV-2.

This book, hopefully, will be more accommodating.

Every disease needs a face—the visage that first registered the illness must be named and memorialised. All too often, that face and name is at several degrees of separation from the origin of the disease—in time and in geography.

When we think of smallpox, we think of Edward Jenner, of the cow-pocked milkmaid Sarah Nelms, of eight-year-old James Phipps and, certainly, of the witty and flamboyant Lady Mary Wortley Montagu. We have no brain-space for the Chinese, Indian and Arab inoculators who were experts in the practice several centuries before Jenner. *We* don't have a face.

When Dr Accacio Viegas astutely diagnosed bubonic plague, a disease previously unknown in Bombay, he failed to record the name of the index patient. Every time I walk past his statue, I reproach him for this.

In 1833, William Twining wrote his classic 200-page treatise on cholera in *The Diseases of Bengal.* His experience of fifteen epidemics of cholera was carefully documented in the book. All his patients were European. 'Asiatics' get honourable mention in one page.

The index patient gives a disease a face, especially when it is as ubiquitous and overwhelming as Covid-19. I had hoped to avoid Dr Viegas's omission, and did what I could to find the medical student who had travelled home to Kasargod from Wuhan. The Kasargod experts were most helpful, but the young man refused an interview. I don't blame him—he should forget the painful experience, and get on with a richly rewarding life. But I would have liked his name, his words, his views in this book.

We are running hard, and we are still fixated on the spot we occupied in 1348 as vantage to a pandemic. I merely choose that year because we have a reliable eyewitness account against which to match our moment:

> I say, then, that such was the energy of the contagion of the said pestilence, that it was not merely propagated from man to man, but, what is much more startling, it was frequently observed, that things which had belonged to one sick or dead of the disease, if touched by some other living creature, not of the human species, were the occasion, not merely of sickening, but of an almost instantaneous death.
>
> In which circumstances, not to speak of many others of a similar or even graver complexion, divers apprehensions and imaginations were engendered in the minds of such as were left alive, inclining almost all of them to the same harsh resolution, to wit, to shun and abhor all contact with the sick and all that belonged to them, thinking thereby to make each his own health secure.

You may argue that *Il Decameron* was a work of fiction, but that was merely because its author, Giovanni Boccaccio, chose this mode of expression to record his observations.

> So marvellous sounds that which I have now to relate, that, had not many, and I among them, observed it with their own eyes, I had hardly dared to credit it, much less to set it down in writing, though I had had it from the lips of a credible witness.

The following passage could be a précis of newspaper accounts from last week, as infection overwhelms many of India's largest metropolises:

> Of the adherents of these divers opinions not all died, neither did all escape; but rather there were, of each sort and in every place, many that sickened, and by those who retained their health were treated after the example which they themselves, while whole, had set, being everywhere left to languish in almost total neglect. Tedious were it to recount, how citizen avoided citizen, how among neighbours was scarce found any that shewed fellow-feeling for another, how kinsfolk held aloof, and never met, or but rarely; enough that this sore affliction entered so deep into the minds of men and women, that in the horror thereof brother was forsaken by brother, nephew by uncle, brother by sister, and oftentimes husband by wife; nay, what is more, and scarcely to be believed, fathers and mothers were found to abandon their own children, untended, unvisited, to their fate, as if they had been strangers. Wherefore the sick of both sexes, whose number could not be estimated, were left without resource but in the charity of friends (and few such there were), or the interest of servants, who were hardly to be had at high rates and on unseemly terms, and being, moreover, one and all, men and women of gross understanding, and for the most part unused to such offices, concerned themselves no further than to supply the immediate and expressed wants of the sick, and to watch them die; in which service they themselves not seldom perished with their gains.

Care is what matters in any illness. Who delivers it? Not the experts who advise the government, nor the oracular mathematicians who cast the planet's daily horoscope, nor even the crack team of mavens who issue protocols and supervise treatment at a digital remove. It is the young doctor, a barely qualified resident, who must deliver the difference between life and death, by quickly placing an IV line, by passing an endotracheal tube, by calming and encouraging the struggling patient. It is the ward boy who must shift gurneys, lift and settle the sick safely from trolley to bed, fix the oxygen mask and offer the bedpan in time. It is the nurse who often does more than the doctor and the ward boy, taking over both their functions with the ease that comes from knowing nobody is there to help.

These vital people, these crucial elements of medical care—they are underpaid and unprotected. Are they not human too? Can you blame them for running away?

Like the 'migrant workers', they have been overlooked in national health policy.

What about domestic policy? Yes, within the home. How do we care for our sick, our aged, our crippled, our incontinent, our confused relations? With loving kindness, one hopes. But lack of resources, information and empathy is a wonderful agar for cruelty.

Domestic cruelty is enshrined in India as a hallowed tradition—irrespective of caste or creed. The victims are always children and the elderly. Women, victims of domineering and brutish patriarchy, themselves perpetuate and nourish its psychopathic machinery.

Through two harrowing years as a resident, when hearing dying declarations from women of my own age burnt to death for dowry, the question, *Who struck the match?* was always answered by the tired whisper: 'She.'

Perhaps we need not continue to mirror the people in Boccacio's narrative. After all, that was 1348. In the interim, if science should have made such great leaps in understanding, we have not been unintelligent. Yet, COVID-19 has ambushed the world in a state of mental déshabillé. We are intellectual and emotional slobs.

We paediatric surgeons are trained with the warning that the scars of our missteps will reproach us for the next hundred years—through a child's lifetime, and long beyond our own. It is a terrible warning, and it reverberates in this time of COVID-19. *Do no harm* is a doctor's first diktat. *Primum non nocere*, because languages like Latin and Sanskrit cut more swagger.

The phrase pounded my skull all of yesterday with migraine-like persistence. I had woken up to the triumphant news of a wonder drug against COVID-19. Feverishly, I accessed the site—and behold, the wonder drug was dexamethasone. It was an old familiar, cheap and accessible. A small trial had shown it reduced deaths in severe cases of COVID-19.

I should have been dancing in jubilation. But all I felt was fear.

Let me explain my dread.

Dexamethasone is a steroid as old as me. Like me, it has seen vicissitudes ecstatically honourable and absolutely horrible. It is a survival drug, used as a last-ditch stand in almost any medical emergency. It may not save a life, but it buys time. And it does that by flooring the brake on inflammation. It can, within minutes, stall, if not reverse, life-threatening inflammation.

It is used in more stable illnesses too. Judiciously, to treat inflammations in a number of chronic diseases. Injudiciously, as a quick fix to hasten a clinical response. Dangerously, as a pep pill, prescribed when the illness has no diagnosis and the prescribing doctor a very tiny brain.

There isn't a doctor alive who hasn't used it some time or another.

And believe you me, there is not a doctor faced with COVID-19 who hasn't reached for this or an allied steroid.

The early COVID-19 story was replete with 'Steroids not recommended' warnings. And now, hey presto, steroids are all we need?

What is a steroid?

The definition I like best is from my old pharmacology textbook: *A patient on steroids can walk all the way to the autopsy room.*

And it is quite literally true. Pumped up on steroids, life feels so good you'd never suspect you're dead. Steroid misusers have long reasoned: Everybody's happy, what's not to like?

In this instance, with dexamethasone being hailed as a wonder drug, several worries cascade:

a. A press release from a politician is a direct message to the public.

b. Dexamethasone tablets are cheap and easily available.

c. In India, where steroids are sold over the counter, people are likely to stockpile and self-medicate.

d. The consequences of popping steroids are disastrous.

Steroids interfere with immunity. That is how they work. That is why they kill.

In this trial, dexamethasone use was confined to patients already so seriously ill that they required a ventilator. Their survival numbers increased. That is a remarkable, even miraculous, finding—even if it isn't strictly news.

Dexamethasone has been used in ARDS in many situations before, with great success. Its place is in the hands of the frontline physician who will use intelligence to administer the drug.

Dexamethasone should NOT be part of a public advisory. Popping steroids can kill.

I take a break—10 a.m. is an unusual time for a walk, but I want to feel the first drizzle. The monsoon has arrived, unperturbed by Cyclone Nisarga's dramatics two weeks ago.

Everybody has forgotten Nisarga already. It is the monsoon we await.

The drizzle is warm as syrup. I almost expect it to taste sweet, but it is a faint fizz on the tongue. Sunlight giggles past the shiny curtain of rain. Everything glitters, clean and burnished. Sparrows chatter. Even crows look less cynical this morning. And then—

I turn the corner and stop, aghast.

I hadn't thought of COVID-19 since I stepped out of the house, but now, in a sudden dazzle of light, I can think, see, feel, nothing else. The strong young rain-tree that spread its canopy across two buildings is missing. The hole in the air is a taut grimace of pain.

The tree has been hacked to pieces—the trunk sawn two feet off the ground, the noble branches chopped into small logs. It was cut not an hour ago. The reek of its injury is still sharp in the air.

The municipality is at its monsoon massacre again. I join the knot of furious residents. Soon, sensible voices have organised a plan of action.

'This is no time to cut trees,' a voice says. I'm a little shocked to recognise it as my own.

'Not with COVID-19. Cases will go up if we cut trees.'

Somebody laughs.

'We can't use that as an excuse,' I'm told kindly. 'There's no connection between trees and COVID.'

They have the natural omniscience of youth. Was I this wise at thirty? Forty? Fifty? Why am I still here?

Suddenly, I find myself talking bats to them. They humour me. They concede the possibility of bats in trees. But the connect between COVID-19 and an invisible bat is a leap of imagination they aren't prepared for. *This* tree, this felled tree and its evicted bats, is what I'm talking about. They are all masked—yet the idea has no takers.

I return dejected, as futile as that tree. How does one notice something hiding in plain sight?

Bocaccio's friend Francesco Petrarch lived through twenty-five years of plague, from his early years as a dandy to his retirement after a stroke to Arquà, where he had a house in the Euganean Hills. The changing vista of the disease was the landscape of his thoughts. He did not chronicle the plague, but followed it inly, permitting it to shape his writing. Standing apart from the sparkling beauty of his poetry is the letter addressed to his soul: *Ad Seipsum* (To Himself).[20] Later, Shelley, who spent his last years in Italy, saw the Euganean Hills as a refuge:

We may live so happy there,
That the Spirits of the Air,
Envying us, may even entice
To our healing paradise
The polluting multitude.[21]

Shelley's poem, *Lines Written Among the Euganean Hills,* carries the emotions of Petrarch's *Letter to Himself*:

> O what has come over me? Where are the violent fates pushing me back to? I see passing by, in headlong flight, time which makes the world a fleeting place. I observe about me dying throngs of both young and old, and nowhere is there a refuge. No haven beckons in any part of the globe, nor can any hope of longed for salvation be seen. Wherever I turn my frightened eyes, their gaze is troubled by continual funerals: the churches groan encumbered with biers, and, without last respects, the corpses of the noble and the commoner lie in confusion

---

20. Francesco Petrarca, *Ad Seipsum* (To Himself), Epistola Metrica I, 14: lines 1–55.
21. Percy Bysshe Shelly, *Lines Written among the Euganean Hills*. 1818.

> alongside each other. The last hour of life comes to mind, and, obliged to recollect my misfortunes, I recall the flocks of dear ones who have departed, and the conversations of friends, the sweet faces which suddenly vanished, and the hallowed ground now insufficient for repeated burials.

Shelley's youthful voice (he was not yet thirty) is one of imagined dread. Petrarch's is the dread of the observer. My own dread. Or yours. It is the momentary paralysis of will we allow ourselves when nothing is expected of us, really, but to keep our heads down and wait it out. It is what the global strategy against COVID-19 has required us to do.

But that momentary paralysis has cost us dear.

It has cost us 3 million lives.

It took six months for science to state what was evident to every clinician worth her or his salt from Day One of this pandemic: *the severity of COVID-19 is one of uncontrolled and uncontrollable inflammation*. Therefore, those who are most vulnerable are those already in a state of inflammation: the elderly, the obese, the undernourished, those with cardiovascular diseases, diabetes, autoimmune diseases. And because this is a respiratory virus, the quality of the air is a deciding factor.

It would have been a simple matter to strategise the lockdown along these lines. By identifying the vulnerable and addressing their vulnerabilities. Some, like the elderly, can only be protected.

The lockdown was a great opportunity for the world to recover its health, but we flubbed it. Policy flubbed it. But we can do better, each one of us.

If you have any of these vulnerabilities, seek medical advice. Get treated. Work at addressing it while you apply simple directives of nutrition, sleep and exercise to optimise your metabolism.

Your doctor will tell you how.

This virus has changed humanity, but how has humanity changed this virus?

From the day it was isolated, scientists have curiously observed changes in SARS-CoV-2. It is the nature of RNA viruses to mutate and mutate fast. What is the implication of these mutations?

Geographic categorisations are iffy. The 'selective sweep' of the D614G mutation across Europe and North America has failed to show any clinical correlation with the severity of the disease. So, too, the finding in Singapore of the 382-nucleotide deletion in ORF8.

Like changes were also observed in SARS-CoV-1. Then, too, there was no correlation between such changes and disease outcomes or transmission rates.

In all, thirty-one mutations have been examined. Do these mutations increase the severity of the disease, make it more infectious or lethal?

No. If at all—and there is a very cautious note of optimism here—these mutations seem to be linked with *reduced* transmissibility. This could explain why, in the early months of the pandemic, India's case load was remarkably low.

'Flattening the curve' is about reducing transmission. A lockdown discourages proximity and so reduces the R_0, the number of people an infected person can infect. It increases the time over which infections double and slows down the epidemic. But there is a fallout. By increasing the duration of the epidemic, it permits the virus to evolve.

The longer a virus circulates in a population, the more distinctive it grows, as mutations accumulate. And we have no idea how this will impact us.

Will this mean new manifestations of COVID-19?

Very possibly.

Will it mean a more lethal form? Or will it mean the disease will subside to a whimper of discomfort, no sooner felt than forgotten?

We must live in hope.

Eventually, this virus, like hundreds of others, will retreat into obscurity to circulate in its reservoirs, uninterested in our species.

The business of capitalism has brought us to this pass by feeding us an industrial diet designed for maximum profit for the few and maximum co-morbidity for the many.

We have fallen into another, perhaps more frightening trap, as a result of this COVID-19 panic. It is the all-pervasive disinfection of the planet. Spraying, wiping, soaking and sluicing everything with disinfectant will make us defenceless against myriad other infections that will come our way tomorrow. Superbugs that will be resistant to all disinfectants, all antibiotics.

Primum non nocere should be the mantra for every decision we take about COVID-19.

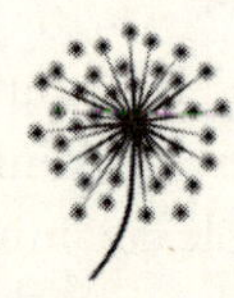

39

The Scum of All Fears

Say a *Homo sapiens*-specific virus—natural or diabolically nano-engineered—picks us off but leaves everything else intact. How would the rest of nature respond if it were suddenly relieved of the relentless pressures we heap on it and our fellow organisms?

– Alan Weisman, *The World Without Us*, 2007

Eventually, pandemics are not about pathogen or disease or death. Pandemics are about the living. About the change in us that determines decisions at global and personal levels. There is universality in our response. The global *is* the personal.

With the spread of COVID-19, our perceptions have regressed to the primitive; our reactions are spring-loaded with dread. Human catapults, we hurl violent injury on each other in the hope that it will save us from this invisible and malignant virus. In the process, unquestioningly, we have allowed the disintegration of human values.

A few months ago, we were stunned by the news that a train had ploughed through sixteen people asleep on the railway tracks near Aurangabad. These were migrant workers walking the 1,000 km journey home. Is it not human to cry out, 'How can we push people to such desperation?' and do our damnedest to keep it from happening again? Or should we ask what I read a week later: *How can anyone stop this when they sleep on railway tracks? There are people walking and not stopping. How can we stop it?*

This was not a nasty bit of snark from a harried householder, scuttling home with his box of mangoes and bottle of sanitiser. It was boomed out from the halls of justice, in answer to the plea that food and shelter were basic entitlements to those on the road.

Cruelty is the new normal. The enemy is no longer the virus. It is the stranger, the neighbour, the family member. Every other human being is now suspect. Viruses could be streaming out of him, straight into your lungs, and who wants that? Kill him, evict him, starve him, torment him and, when he's dead, throw his body to the dogs and shoot the dogs.

Not an extreme scenario. Incidents not far from this, too painful to recall here, have made the news. The invariable comment is: *But what can people do?*

That is not a rhetorical question. It demands answers deeper than the directives of social distancing, masking and disinfection.

Cruelty and violence are signs of despair and ignorance. The terror of loss erases reason. And world over, governments have authorised panic:

Be afraid, be very afraid!

As of 5 July, COVID-19 has claimed 528,204 lives. In India, the number of cases has climbed to 697,412, with 19,693 deaths. The US, the worst affected so far, has lost 129,576 lives.

The pundits tell us every day: 'So many more would have died without these measures.' They may be right. Or not. When all else fails, there is always statistics.

This is not a war against a malignant virus. The war is within us.

The battle might be within our lungs, true, but isn't it time we noticed this is a larger war?

Pandemics are silly season for conspiracy theories. My inbox is flooded with earnest harangues about lab-engineered viruses, mind control, 5G and hatewrite against every other neighbourhood / nation / religion / food habits / language, things you never even imagined could engender a killer virus. The delete button on my keyboard is getting worn out, but I still miss an old favourite among terrors: panspermia. The term was invented by the fifth-century Greek polymath Anaxagoras,[22] when he decided that meteors were bits of larger stars. He predicted that if the heavenly bodies should be loosened by some slip or shake, one of them might be torn away, and might plunge and fall down to earth. And, with it, carry seeds everywhere, thus generating life. Aristotle pipped him at the post with the more believable spontaneous generation of life.

Forgotten for nearly 2,000 years, Anaxagoras was revived at the turn of the nineteenth century. His theory that life rained down from outer space has quietly grown stronger. Things took a serious turn when astrobiology became a respectable science. Fred Hoyle and Chandra Wickramasinghe published *Diseases from Space* in 1979. They ascribed the 1918 flu pandemic to an unspecified extraterrestrial source. It did not go down well. After the SARS epidemic of 2003, the idea was revived briefly—as it will be now, without doubt.

The Indian Space Research Organisation has conducted air-sampling balloon experiments for a long time. In 2009, three novel strains of bacteria were recovered from altitudes of 27 and 41 km. They were named *Janibacter hoylei* sp. nov., in honour of Fred Hoyle; *Bacillus isronensis* sp. nov.; and *Bacillus aryabhattai* sp. nov.

What were these bacteria doing up there? They were chance encounters in the stratosphere, probably curiosities, nothing more.

---

22. Anaxagoras, 'Lord of the Assembly', c.510–c.428 BCE. My favourite line of his is: *The descent to hell is the same from every place.*

How do germs travel? Viruses that are genetically identical are often discovered great distances apart, in different habitats. We know how quickly viruses change their genomes to adapt to new environments. And yet, two sets of an identical genome may thrive in starkly different habitats. That could happen if the virus had a host with a very wide range, like a bird or a human jet-traveller. Or if it were dispersed by a very long-armed natural agency. Wind, or water.

The atmosphere is divided into the troposphere (extending 7 miles up from the earth's surface) and, 30 miles beyond, the stratosphere. The stratosphere, long imagined as pristine, allows unimpeded transit of anything wafted up there. In the troposphere, there is a mixing of suspended particles. We simply presumed that when they fall to earth, they would do so locally.

Curtis Suttle of British Columbia examines the distribution of viruses in nature. Suttle's group sampled air from 1.7 km above sea level in the Sierra Nevada mountains in Spain. The air samples had intrusions from Saharan dust storms and from the Westerlies over the Atlantic. They found an incredible number of viruses and bacteria in the sampled air.

There were more viruses than bacteria [109/m^2/day as compared to 106/m^2/day]. Viruses were attached to the smallest airborne organic particles [< 0.7 microns] and so stayed up for much longer than bacteria which had hooked up with larger aerosols.

After a long sojourn in the troposphere, viruses can fall on the earth's surface at sites that are far removed from their places of origin.

At any point in time, millions of viruses rain down on us, are blown past us, settle on us, are swallowed by us and, yes, are inhaled and exhaled by us.

If all the 1×10^{31} viruses on earth were laid end to end, they would stretch for 100 million light years.

Physical distancing?

Hahaha.

I have looked at the first stirrings of this disease in Wuhan. I've looked at it from the lung's point of view. I have looked at it from the vantage of the virus. I've examined the body of evidence from the autopsy slab. I've considered its origins in bats. All this, and I'm still short of the quintessential COVID-19. I know the plot, but I need the narrative entire.

And then, through a chance phone call, I hear it.

The phone slides from my trembling hand. The voice at the other end keeps speaking. I wait for it to cease. In the silence, I watch the story unfold.

I might have met Dinesh at some point. He was one of the boys who worked in an eatery, perhaps one of the many down my road. I might have caught a glimpse of him slathering a pau with butter and balancing it on a volcanic surge of bhaji. Or slicing onions, wristing the knife with samurai speed. Or dipping dishes in a pail of murky water. Or shooting the breeze on the pavement with his pals. Or, maybe, I never met him at all.

But there he is, indistinguishable in the crowd of young men, intent in stride towards the highway.

Dinesh's eatery, like the rest of them on this road, downed its shutters a month ago. He was let go with but a semblance of severance pay.

Others had it worse: they had been turned out without a pice. Still, the money wouldn't even see the week through. He had to pay for food and shelter.

Dinesh called home. 'Stay where you are,' his father answered nervously. 'You'll find work.'

'There's no work here. Everything's shut down.'

'You'll manage.'

Dinesh stuck it out for a fortnight. He banded with a group of guys from his neck of the woods, and here they were. His backpack contained his uniform, carefully folded. A towel. A new T-shirt he had saved for his younger brother. A bottle of water. A packet of chips. Travel light, his companions advised, we'll find food on the way.

And so they did, at first, when the going was still a trek, a picnic, a chancy adventure. They hitched rides when they could, but these were short stretches on the 350 km journey to Pandharpur.

How long did the journey take?

Long enough for Dinesh to retch with hunger and turn giddy with heat and exhaustion. Brief enough for his heart to rejoice at the thought of home.

It was late afternoon when he reached the village. The pagdandi that led off the highway seemed to go on and on, and when he finally glimpsed the turning that led into the hamlet, he broke into a run.

For the first time he felt the breeze in his dusty hair, the power in his legs and a song in his heart, as he let fly the piercing whistle he knew his brother would recognise.

When he turned the corner he found a crowd scattered in the patches of shade. Their sullen exhaustion stopped his thudding feet.

Somebody had died.

His guts tightened in anxiety and, fearfully, he hurried.

Nobody had died.

The crowd, which now absorbed him in its silence, was barricaded from the village. The bamboo fence wasn't much of a deterrent. Despite the barbed wire looping across, it could be easily crossed.

The deterrents stood on the other side, rods and staves in hand. Their turbans were wound tight over their faces, but what could be seen of them looked familiar.

Dinesh addressed them by name.

The answer was swift and terse.

The staves were jabbed in his direction.

They could have been staving off a mad dog, for their feet retreated in a nervous shuffle as their shoulders moved, their faces turned away.

'They won't hear a word,' someone spoke angrily. 'None of us are sick. Are you?'

'Do I look sick?' Dinesh shot back. 'I've walked all the way from Mumbai.'

One by one bitter voices surged, with competing stories of hardship.

'Why won't they let us in if we aren't sick?' Dinesh protested.

'It's the quarantine.'

'So where are we supposed to wait?'

'Here. Or go back.'

'They'll send us food, won't they?'

It was a wasted question. They had been waiting, hungry, since yesterday.

Dinesh called home. A computerised voice said the number he was trying to reach had been switched off.

Night fell.

Dinesh had begged and bribed a guard to carry home news of his arrival.

New guards arrived. They carried flash lamps, LED lanterns brighter than any he had seen before.

He gave himself an hour, no two, for his brother to come hurrying up to pull him in past the barricade. His father would come too, and give these guards a kick or two. He may be old, but he was still the wrestler who had trained these louts.

'I'll get you home,' he assured the crowd. 'My father will be here soon.'

They answered with silence.

Dinesh paced the path. It was no use waiting at the barricade. Each time he approached, the guards thrust their staves at him.

Clarity returned to Dinesh. Journey forgotten, in that instant he became the canny village teenager he was.

Melting into the shadows, he crept his way out through the bushes, swishing his backpack to frighten away snakes. He found the path he remembered. It circled the village and led to the ruined factory beyond—that would be unguarded, for sure.

It was.

Dinesh took off his shoes and walked barefoot through the sleeping village. It was past midnight when he reached home.

He ran up the path he had got paved the last time he was home. He ran up the steps he scrubbed out every morning he was home. And here he was, at the door.

He wanted to shout out, 'Ai, Baba, I'm here!'

But even his knock was muted. His heartbeat was louder by far.

He knocked again.

He had been waiting a lifetime, he had been waiting a trice, when lights came on.

He heard his father's heavy approach.

The door opened.

His father's burly frame filled the doorway. He caught a glimpse of his mother beyond.

Why so dull, so anxious? So drained of welcome? What had happened?

A sudden fear gripped him. He cried out his brother's name—

Before the word had died on the air, they disappeared, Baba and Ai.

Dinesh was left facing the stubborn door.

It had bruised his nose in its slam.

Feet retreated.

Lights went out.

The village slept.

It would have been easy for Dinesh to scale the water-pipe and get to the terrace. He could have hooted like an owl, the signal his brother knew so well. Surely it would rouse him and his skinny arms would pull Dinesh into the warm bed.

But Dinesh did not do that.

He was magnetised in sudden understanding.

He moved swiftly, with a sureness of purpose he had lacked till now.

There was no time to waste, he told himself. He checked the clock on his phone. It was 1 a.m.

In a few minutes, he had found what he was looking for. Dinesh walked towards the temple.

The temple was small for this village, but big enough for the Deva. Every time the Deva granted a prayer, villagers strung up another bell to add to the daily clamour.

There were more bells than the rope slung across the door could sustain.

Much against his will, on his last visit, Dinesh had coughed up cash for the strong steel rod that now took the weight of those bells.

It had been a good investment, after all. The rod gleamed in the dark. There was space for a dozen bells more.

And, surely, space enough for him.

The village rose late. It was eight before they called the police.

When the police got there at eleven, they found the villagers had already acted.

A bamboo fence enclosed the temple. Men armed with rods and staves ringed the fence. What were they prepared to fight?

Why, the most recent answer to their prayers, now hanging between the silent bells.

When I had dropped the phone, I heard the voice of my friend continue the story.

The police had taken away Dinesh's body and cremated it far away from the village.

His backpack had been cremated too. His father had insisted on it, after the police confirmed it contained no cash.

Dinesh's story is so common that it has lost meaning. There are too many like Dinesh to be granted identity, and too few for statistics.

Yet Dinesh's story encapsulates the story of Covid-19, and its meaning must be recovered, in all its layers of dread.

To all semblance, Dinesh's family did the right thing by society. They protected the village and, quite incidentally, themselves. They are pitied, perhaps revered, as parents who made the supreme sacrifice. They typify the face of altruism. Soon, eulogised, memorialised, deified, they will become legend.

Myths mushroom in the sunless spaces of survival. Nothing else will grow here except bizarre rationalisations of the irrational. For it *is* irrational for a parent to reject a child.

I'm quite sure if Dinesh's parents were to speak about the moment of slamming the door on their son, they would recall it as *doing our duty*.

Duty is the fig leaf that hides our shame. Rip it away, and what's exposed?

An undervalued and very expressive body part.

The thinking brain.

We are ashamed to express doubt and uncertainty.

Fearful of questions, we deny the truth, and quickly grab at the nearest duty as uniform.

Now we may breathe easy.

Unnoticed in the faceless crowd, now we may, with a bit of luck, survive.

Dinesh's parents committed no crime. In their eyes, Dinesh, coming from an infected city, carried instant death. What if the village caught the virus? Would they not be guilty of mass murder? They exculpated that unthinkable enormity by slamming the door on their son. They are not responsible for what happened after that. They did the best they could, and no one can do more.

Oh, but I think we can.

I begin by looking at three levels of meaning in Dinesh's story, through keener eyes than mine.

I step outside, masked as required, shopping bag dangled as insignia of purpose, swift of pace, fearful of my neighbours.

They are queued six feet apart for fruit or vegetables they will doubtless scrub with soap, steep in disinfectant, peel with a sterilised knife, autoclave or incinerate, and slip in sideways past the mask, using disposable cutlery.

I notice there is only one commodity guaranteed virus-proof. Nobody's actually admitted it, but as Jane would have said, it is a truth universally acknowledged. Cash alone is above contagion.

I'm devious this morning. My shopping bag is camouflage. I'm here to look, not buy. The empty stretch of road is familiar—not because I live here but because all empty streets look the same. I need to see this COVID-19 exterior past the mirage of the familiar, and the eyes I choose are de Chirico's.

Giorgio de Chirico, with *pittura metafisica*, documented his long present in the shadow of the mythic past. He painted turbulence recollected in stillness, cityscapes of empty buildings, abandoned lots spring-loaded with violence. Fractured sculptures and classical artefacts witness the passage of time, depicted as speeding trains. His paintings are supple narratives of the velocity of vanishing and the persistence of being. They form the external landscape of COVID-19. I will pick just one: *Le Chant d'amour*, or *The Song of Love*, painted in 1914. It could be an approximate illustration of Dinesh's particular story.

For its sculptural element, *The Song of Love* has the classical head of an ephebe, a young Greek of Dinesh's age, displayed on a dun brown windowless wall. Nailed in place next to it is a gigantic surgical glove, wetly gleaming, as if recently stripped off.

The glove radiates menace. The beautiful head offers helplessness, passivity. Around them the city is an ingemination of arches, walling off the unexplored depth of emptiness. In contrapunct to this stolid fixity, a ball has rolled into the foreground. Eerily lit by an unseen source at the lower right of the frame, its green is the perfect complement to the red glove.

All this while the train has been speeding … any minute now the ball will roll away.

The emptiness threatens with the unstated. The destiny of the virus, terrible, inevitable. The conjunction of helplessness and discipline, meant to protect, make up a rigid geometry of control. Against this menace, the architecture of arches and clean angles is soothing, with its promise of shelter and safety.

What is the interior landscape of that safe home?

I turn to Edward Hopper, the portraitist of alienation. His solitary figures conceal their stories. Very few reveal their features, and yet their bodies confess an embattled spirit. We long to engage them, but they ignore us.

Every painting of Hopper's—even his landscapes and interiors without people—exclude the viewer. The fall of a shutter is very nearly audible.

The girl in *Compartment C Car 293* (1938) has a book open in her lap, but we know at once she isn't really reading. She is keeping up that pretence to shield her bubble of loneliness. It should have been a cosy scene—a comfortable seat in a lit nook, winged scenery at the window, the colours a restful palette of olive green.

But it isn't.

Her isolation makes of the nook a cell. Her pretence at reading conceals a powerful upheaval she must shield at all costs from the viewer. What distress is she fleeing from? What pain awaits her? The painting is a brilliant juxtaposition of certainty and anxiety.

The interior landscape of Covid-19 is that of the home we carry within us, the rooms we inhabit alone and refuse to share. Hopper's *Sun in an Empty Room* (1963) is that space. We descend to that sunlit floor, back against the wall. Captive by circumstance, passive in un-choice, we make deals with ourselves to see this time through.

How will we emerge?

How will this climate of fear and uncertainty warp us?

This brings me to Picasso's *Self Portrait On Facing Death* (1972). It is like looking into the mirror, although that isn't what the mirror shows me. It is the totality of dread, reduced to a few simple lines of colour. The spirit bleeds from the unequal pulsatile eyes. Neither unfleshed bone nor creased old age, it is the nakedness of despair.

Dinesh's story is our story too. We are included in the script not because we inflict cruel rejections or succumb to terror and despair, but because we perceive the virus as an invisible enemy in ceaseless pursuit, one that we can effectively shut out by a few simple rules.

A social species embracing the unsocial, we overlook how our world is being reshaped as we hunker down at home.

Fear is human, even productive, as it spurs us to heights of imagination and discovery. But panic is the scum of all fears, choking the oxygen out of us long before any virus can.

A witty punster sent me this yesterday:

Q: What's the difference between Covid-19 and *Romeo and Juliet*?

A: *One's a corona virus, the other a crisis in Verona.*

It reminded me that *Romeo and Juliet* was Shakespeare's vision of the plague. Not just the curse that resounds through every line: *A plague on both your houses!*

The Bard had much to say about isolation and brooding too. Here is Macbeth cogitating on the verge of murder:

But now I am cabined, cribbed, confined, bound in
To saucy doubts and fears.

Those very doubts and fears scum our immured thoughts these days with malevolence.

What we are—our immune system, our memory, our cognition—are legacies of ancient infections. Eight per cent of our genome is testimony to this. Every time we get a viral infection, an iota of viral material is absorbed into our genome.

Life without viruses is impossible. Perhaps life itself is possible because of viruses. Which is why our strategies against this one should be directed more towards our response to infection. I'm not talking therapies and vaccines here, those are on the way, and cannot be hurried. They are being brilliantly invented, carefully tested and judiciously used. Frontline physicians are stretched beyond endurance and are still unfailingly compassionate and introspective. I'm talking about we, the huddle. How can we get equipped to deal with the virus *if we're infected*?

Is there anything, anything at all, we can do to reduce the incidence of the fatal complications of COVID-19? Today, these are no longer confined to ARDS. There are neurological, cardiac and renal terrors too. Above all, the threat to children is on the increase. We still don't know if the virus is sexually transmissible, and whether it can affect the unborn. The bottom line? Anything is possible.

Our response so far has been the ancient riposte of slamming the door on the enemy. Testing is chancy. Yes, an asymptomatic person may cough, sneeze, even breathe out viruses, and that person is very likely to be me or you or anyone else. Very likely, the virus is already an accepted member of the human virome.

What then? How can we be certain we won't die from it?

We can't, but we do have a few observations to go by:

~ The significance of a positive PCR test in the absence of symptoms is vexed. A positive test can mean you've recently been ill or that you may soon be ill. But there also is evidence that such mucosal infections begin, persist and terminate in the absence of symptoms.

~ The billion-dollar question of course: *Is such a person infectious?* Viral infections are a constant state. If we were to examine the mucosal surfaces of the entire population on the planet for viral particles by RT-PCR, we would come up with a staggeringly high incidence of 'dangerous viruses' in apparently healthy people. What should we do then? In that case, the presence of the virus in apparently healthy people wouldn't matter in the least—unless they infect others.

~ And these others may simply accept the virus as part of 'normal' flora, and remain asymptomatic. That is, unless they go into the inflammatory response that leads to ARDS.

So, any how we look at it, the crucial need is to prevent the uncontrolled inflammatory response.

Can we do that?

We can only try to control or prevent aggravating factors.

The clinical pictures from various countries inform us that the worst outcomes are in people who have associated illnesses with inflammatory profiles. High on this list is obesity. Diabetes and cardiovascular illnesses follow as a consequence.

The link between particulate air pollution and inflammatory changes in the lung is undeniable.

These factors can be addressed urgently, not just at the personal level but as a societal strategy to control Covid-19.

Such an approach will quarrel with the strategy so firmly in place now.

Limitation of physical space is the Indian reality. Only 1 per cent of the populace has adequate living space. Physical proximity will act as an incubator for disease, any disease, not just this one.

'Social distancing' has been a spectacular success in India for over 3,000 years. It has produced a fissured and prejudiced society that fragments under stress. The caste system is our greatest vulnerability as much as it is our deepest shame. The Indian Constitution is a remarkable attempt to overturn these injustices and restore equity of purpose and harmony to our society. It should be required reading, lest we emerge from COVID-19 with a new, and even more injurious and fragmentary, caste system.

In poor, over-crowded countries like India and Brazil, physical distancing is purely illusory. Most crowded housing areas, not just slums, become hotbeds of disease because of the enforced proximity. Add to this the consequent lack of physical activity and the compulsive eating of packaged, processed and snack foods. Compound this with the concentration of cooking fumes in a confined space, local incineration of waste, dust from vacant constructions sites and abandoned projects, and there is enough to explain the AQI of 392 in Bombay in the midst of the lockdown—a period *without vehicular traffic and with padlocked factories.*

This, surely, can be addressed at the policy level?

At the individual level, much more can be achieved. Reorienting our perception to COVID-19 will restore in us a sense of responsibility towards our health. Right now, it is limited to mask-and-scrub, a near-Pavlovian response.

As I wrote that last line, almost as if gnomes were reading my brain, in pinged an offer to sell me a plastic shield. A mask is now mandatory lingerie, but this clear, rigid, plastic cylinder will wall me in from temple to clavicles. Barely had I digested this when a friend called because he needed PPE to travel on a train. Masked and gloved though he would be, the virus was likely to encrust the rest of him without a protective bodysuit that would give him heatstroke in minutes.

Another ping. A Darth Vader N95, I guessed. People are 3-D printing them like crazy. Add that to PPE, and you have Doctor Schnabel, circa 2020.

Dr Schnabel held a nosegay too. Perhaps that will become a diagnostic aid now: *Can't smell a rose? Isolate!*

Vos Creditis, als eine Fabel, quod scribitur vom Doctor Schnabel? demands the macaronic legend on the portrait of Dr Schnabel: *Did you think this was a fable written by Dr Schnabel?*

The strange apparition in the portrait has the fantastic guise of a lesser Egyptian deity, Europeanised with a hat. A bird head with a most definite beak. He is dressed in a cumbrous floor-length robe. His hands suggest tough gloves. He steps with caution, and he brandishes a stick. In the background, alarmed figures flee his approach.

Our Dr Schnabel is less self-assured. His fable is being written by the Schrödinger virus—equally present and absent at any given time—and so must continue to baffle and mystify.

Why not reclaim the playbook?

Why not reconsider Covid-19 from the human vantage, from *our* point of view?

And while we wait for vaccines and therapies, why not repair health?

Whose life is it, anyway?

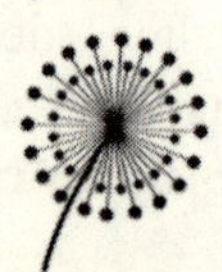

The blackboard is erased in the attic
And the wind turns up the light of the stars,
Sinewy now. Someone will find out, someone will know.
And if somewhere in this great planet
The truth is discovered, a patch of it, dried, glazed by the sun,
It will just hang on, in its own infamy, humility. No one
Will be better for it, but things can't get any worse.
Just keep playing, mastering as you do the step
Into disorder this one meant. Don't you see
It's all we can do? Meanwhile, great fires
Arise, as of haystacks aflame. The dial had been set
And that's ominous, but all your graciousness in living
Conspires with it, now that this is our home:
A place to be from, and have people ask about.

– John Ashberry, *Rain Moving In*, 1983

'Like all great stories, COVID-19 is a tragedy, a love story gone seriously wrong.'

As COVID-19 sweeps the planet, we are panicked and baffled. Bombarded with disinformation and panic-inducing statistics, we are cowed by the enormity and uncertainty of what's unfolding.

The narrative, so far, has been about this novel coronavirus.

But COVID-19 is not just about SARS-CoV-2.

It is about the virus and us.

We have coexisted with viruses from the dawn of evolution. What has changed? Is it this 'new virus'? Or, has something changed in us? Have we disrupted something crucial in Nature?

A Crown of Thorns is science and history woven into the human story—the long view on a pandemic that's consuming us.

Drs Ishrat Syed and Kalpana Swaminathan, writing as Kalpish Ratna, distil their study of plagues and epidemics into a work packed with ideas that provoke and insights that illuminate.

The clearest account yet of COVID-19, this book will endure new revelations about this virus and serve as a strong basis for future understanding.